Awaken Wellness

Awaken Wellness

How to Navigate Through the Hell of Chronic Illness and Heal Your Life

Dion Murtagh

Copyright © 2016 by Dion Murtagh. All rights reserved

No part of this publication may be reproduced, distributed, or transmitted in any form or by any means, including photocopying, recording, or other electronic or mechanical methods, without the prior written permission of the publisher, except in the case of brief quotations embodied in critical reviews and certain other noncommercial uses permitted by copyright law.

The information contained in this book is not intended to serve as a replacement for medical advice. Any use of the information in this book is at the reader's discretion. The author is not a doctor. He presents an overview of what helped on his personal journey to recovery from severe chronic fatigue syndrome through his own learning, application of knowledge and self-experimentation when the medical profession either couldn't or wouldn't help. This book is an overview of this personal knowledge and is not intended to replace medical testing or medical diagnosis. Professional and peer advice should always be sought before undertaking any manner of detox, supplement, dietary, psychological or exercise program. The author specifically disclaims any and all liability arising directly or indirectly from the use or application of any information contained in this book.

For my girls, my lights through the darkness.

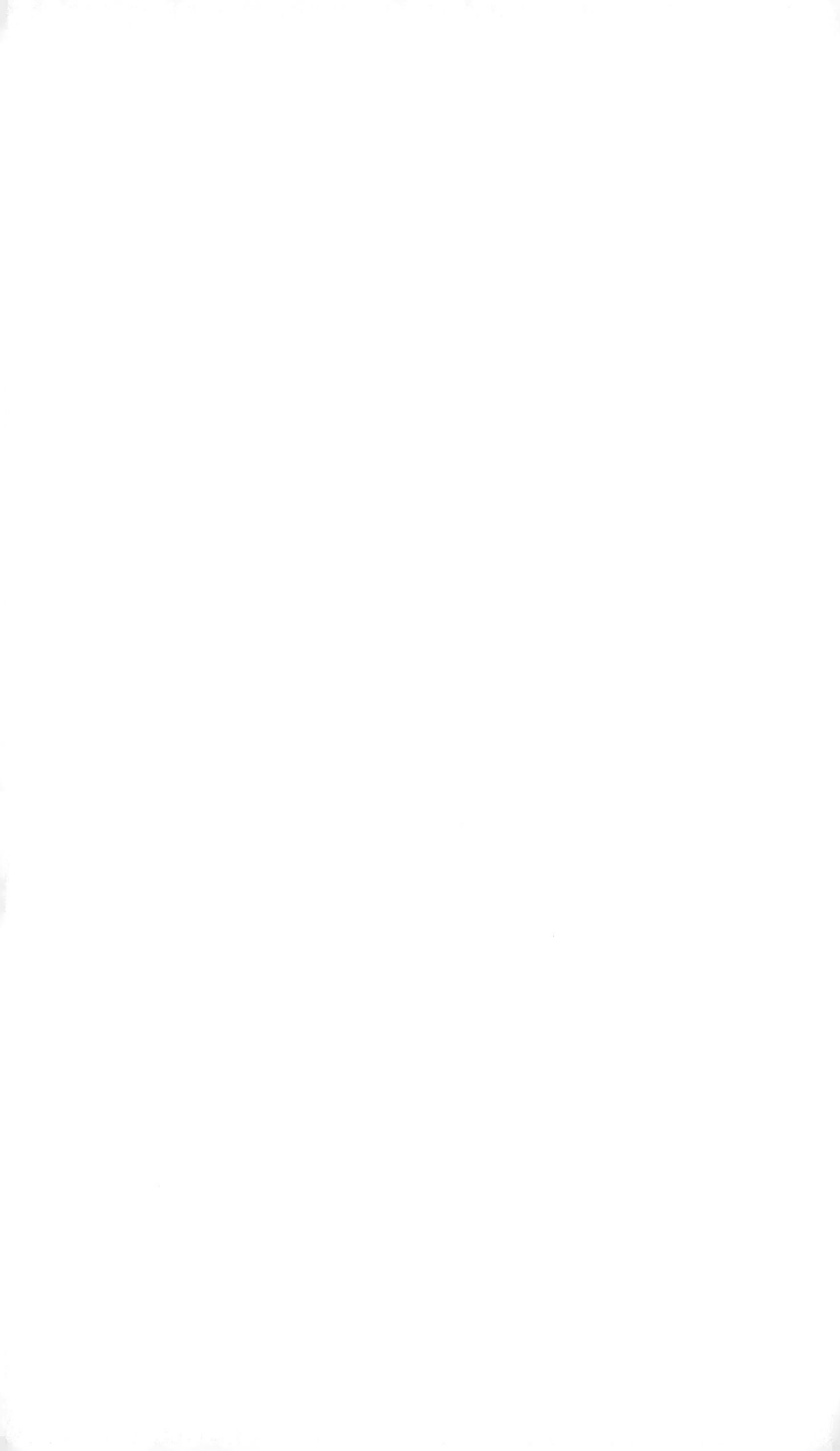

Contents

Introduction	15
What's in a Name?	17
The Instant Descent	19
"I" Was Gone	22
Abandoned in a Broken System	24
The Thriving Sickness Business	28
The University of Google	31
CFS Schools of Thought	33
The Roadblocks	37
Patients: The New Authority	40
To the Healthy Person	44
Become Your Own Guinea Pig	47
The Broken Body	**49**
The Broken Body	50
Know Your Past, Heal Your Future	55
The Virus Myth–Which Came First?	58
Healing the Broken Body	60
Enjoying Pacing	62
Take Out the Trash!	65
Who Pulled the Plug?	67
Nutrition: Healing the Second Brain	69
Gluten: the Inflammatory Monster	71
Going Organic vs Eating Glycophosphates	72
Avoid Processed Sugars	74
Eat Every 2.5 Hours	76
Cortisol and the Gut	77
Fat is Your Friend	78
Good Bugs	79
Supplements	81
Healthy Sleep	93

Testing: The Hidden Factors	98
Gut Integrity	107
The MTHFR of a Mutation!	110
Chiropractic Care	112
Bounce!	114
Cold Shower Therapy	115
The Broken Brain	**117**
The Broken Brain	118
The Physiology of Emotional Stress	120
Healing the Broken Brain	123
Reframing the Stress Response	125
Hold Nothing Back	128
Mickel Therapy	132
The Initially Terrifying Act of Not Resting!	136
Rewiring the Idiot Driver	139
Listen to Your Symptoms	141
The Switch Had Been "Flipped"	144
Energy Vampires	148
Epigenetics	150
Meditation	152
Emotional Freedom Technique	155
The Power of Expectation	159
Positive Psychology	161
The Broken Spirit	**164**
The Broken Spirit	165
Healing the Broken Spirit	168
The Art of Flourishing	170
Family	174
The Ocean	177
Life in Increments	179
Waiting to Live	181
Art as Therapy	183
Gratitude	186

Never Stop Learning	188
Mindfulness	190
Wise Attention	195
Qi Gong	197
Visualisation	199
Affirmations	203
PMA	207
The Three Difficulties	209
Claiming Your Power	210
Resilient Thinking	212
Mastery	216
Love is All	218
I Am Grateful for Chronic Fatigue Syndrome	221
Thank you	223

The medicine for my suffering I had within me from the very beginning, but I did not take it.
My ailment came from within myself, but I did not observe it until this moment.
Now I see that I will never find the light unless, like a candle, I am my own fuel.
—Bruce Lee

"I was given a one page info sheet and told by my doctor Chronic Fatigue Syndrome was forever and I should just go home to bed. So I did. For over a year. I couldn't read, write, speak, shower myself, cook, lift my arms or walk, and lived with constant agonizing pain, tinnitus, migraines, and brain fog. I developed allergic reactions to foods and smells, and merely existed, requiring no light and sound to survive the hours.

"I was told to accept this fate, but refused. I had to educate myself, fight for tests and argue with doctors who laughed in my face, but I persevered. I took small compounding actions every single day for years.

"Now I am well. And I fight for you."

—Dion Murtagh.

Introduction

Introduction

This is a book of healing and empowerment. It is a guide of hope for the hopeless. It is my journey through hell with severe Chronic Fatigue Syndrome to recovery and thriving wellness. I will not say "to hell and back", for that implies I returned to my old self. I am an entirely new person: healthy, vibrant, unconquerable. This book gives a voice to the voiceless, suffering as I was with unimaginable torment, ignored, discarded, and abandoned by the wider medical profession for being afflicted with a condition they do not understand and many won't even acknowledge.

I believe this book to be vital in encompassing a complete and holistic mind-body-spirit approach to self-healing from Chronic Fatigue Syndrome. It was born from my own recovery process and a desire to share my story, knowing the same level of healing I have experienced is possible to anyone with the right guidance. The fact is, there is no guidance or help from the system CFS sufferers entrust with and wait upon for a solution to this seemingly incurable chronic illness. Healing is up to you and the resource you need is in your hands. Although pertaining to CFS, this book is valuable for anyone going through ANY chronic illness right now, as well as the carers of those affected. This isn't just a book about good food or positive thinking. You cannot wish CFS away. As you know CFS is a complex biological beast of an illness, but when it comes down to it, sometimes the most multifaceted of problems have the simplest solutions, when these are combined and applied correctly.

You will learn how to literally undo, unravel and rebuild yourself from a lifetime of viral infections, inflammation, physical trauma, poor food choices, environmental toxicity, pharmaceuticals, gut damage, cellular damage, perfectionism, emotional stress and metabolic imbalances. Healing from CFS requires attentively bringing many factors into harmony. It is simple once you make a choice to heal yourself, but it's not entirely easy and will take dedication to maintain optimal health for the rest of your life.

This book will be your catalyst to create a complete shift in your being, allowing you to heal on a deep cellular level. You will unfasten entangled physical blocks and obstructive emotional patterns that may have limited you throughout your life as you nourish and empower yourself back to health. You will awaken to a new joy every single day, as you gradually begin to experience a release from the hell that CFS confines you to. I encourage you to give everything to this journey. If you are where I was, besieged every minute with agonizing symptoms, then you really have nothing to lose. Give this book your full attention and you will be blessed with knowing you have developed the resources inside to heal yourself and live the life you want. And best of all, YOU will have done it yourself. The answers lie within.

What's in a Name?

What's in a Name?

For the purposes of universality, I have maintained the most widely used name, Chronic Fatigue Syndrome (CFS), created in 1994 as a case definition by researchers struggling to understand something that still wasn't even acknowledged as an illness. In 2015, the US Institute of Medicine renamed CFS "Systemic Exertion Intolerance Disease" (SEID) which, like "CFS", grossly understates the complex nature of the illness and only isolates one characteristic. The label frequently used in the UK is Myalgic Encephalomyelitis (ME), but this in itself only refers to the inflammatory aspect of the brain and central nervous system. People like to argue that one is worse than the other, that CFS is 'not as severe' as ME and that nobody ever recovers from either. It's all labels and none of them bring sufferers any closure, solutions or lights at the end of the long, dark tunnel of chronic illness. The labels make no difference whatsoever to governments, or within the world's medical research fraternity, especially given the fact people are now crowd funding to raise research dollars, due to the lack of government funding for treating the illness. To illustrate my point, research into curing male pattern baldness secures three times more government funding annually in the US than research for Chronic Fatigue Syndrome, despite there being over 3 million diagnosed sufferers of the illness. The undiagnosed are innumerable.

Whether you wish to label yourself as having CFS, ME, SEID, or whatever newly coined name pops out of someone's research paper in the coming years, the fact is it's all horrible to varying degrees in every single individual. Arguing over one's chronic illness label does not bring you any closer to healing yourself from it. Therefore, the name is basically irrelevant, aside from the fact that a not-as-serious sounding name like Chronic Fatigue Syndrome isn't afforded the credibility by ignorant medical professionals as something with the more clinical-sounding name, Myalgic Encephalomyelitis. I say this from personal experience, having used both names during encounters with doctors, as a sociological experiment to gauge their reactions and subsequent standard of treatment. For argument's sake, let's just all agree it is hell to live with!

The Instant Descent

The Instant Descent

My journey through hell started when I was 37. Actually, a multitude of contributing factors meant I was fatigued and struggling daily in secret and well on my way to chronic illness for many years before then, but I'll discuss the details of that later. The instant descent, though, was fast and brutal. One sunny day, I went with my family to check out an art exhibition and was feeling a little off. Upon entering the gallery, I felt apprehensive and confused, as the lights in the room seemed to be flickering and the noise of the visitors was overwhelming my senses. Anxiety and unease that something was wrong crept over me. Within 20 minutes I was in full blown panic, feeling faint and nauseous, and I knew I had to get out of there, thinking I was maybe having a panic attack or rapidly coming down with some kind of virus. I went home to bed and didn't get up for two weeks.

Those weeks were spent hallucinating, along with tinnitus, migraines, fevers, glands swollen like grapes and a body that felt like it had been beaten from the inside out with a bat. I was barely able to move, the whole time thinking 'this is the worst virus I've ever had.' I eventually got myself to the doctor, who said my ears were inflamed and prescribed antibiotics. After a couple more weeks of this bedridden state, I had a clear morning, so I was determined to at least get out of the house and go for a walk. I went for a 15-minute walk and felt extremely lethargic, but not sick. I was glad to be out of bed, but instinctively felt something still wasn't right.

That evening I was right back where I'd started! Migraines, tinnitus, burning muscles and joints! It was hell. The doctor ordered a range of blood tests this time and sent me home with more antibiotics. After a week or so I returned to the doctor, who said my bloods were all clear and normal. As I'd experienced a lot of recurring fatigue, pain and 'viruses' for years prior to this, she took me through a series of diagnostic questions and hit me with the news I have Chronic Fatigue Syndrome. I asked what it involves and how long until I'm better, to which she replied, "some people never recover. You need to go home and stay in bed. No more physical training or stress." She handed me a one-page health department sanctioned printout on CFS that was apparently all the information I needed to manage living life with CFS. I think I left there in shock, and it wasn't until I got home and mentally struggled through an hour of Internet research of my own that I realised the gravity of the condition I was facing. I remember thinking at the time, "if I was diagnosed with cancer, at least I'd either die or be cured." With CFS, it seemed it was going to be complete uncertainty forever. I felt like my life was over.

The next two months were spent pretty much the same as the previous – in bed, struggling to cope with the symptoms. I couldn't sleep at all. I was so tired, but wired with racing thoughts and constant migraines. I could barely lift a fork or spoon to my mouth, and began to develop food intolerances and allergies. Any scent of perfume or cleaning product sent my system into panic, bordering on anaphylactic response. I had to be in complete darkness and silence, as anything else was sensory overload.

Being almost unable to move, walk, speak, listen and feed or

The Instant Descent

shower myself had become my new reality. Some days it took all of my will and energy to simply take another breath. Then another. Then another. It felt like my lungs were filled with concrete and every cell and nerve in my body was on fire, right through to my toes. Seconds felt like hours in this unbelievably excruciating fatigue. When you barely have the energy to take your next breath, you start to think things you wouldn't normally. There were times I wished I would just die so I didn't have to face another minute like that. Those endless minutes went on for years.

"I" Was Gone

Only a few months earlier, I was an aspiring entrepreneur, a writer, artist, musician, amateur photographer with a love of the ocean, road trips, mountain biking, bushwalking and reading, and a thirst for knowledge in health, nutrition, psychology, exercise science and martial arts. I was, at 37, the fittest I'd ever been in my life, loved lifting heavy weights and sprint training and living on mostly organic food. Despite various "mystery illnesses" repeatedly knocking me down for a decade, I was an active and joyful dad and husband, the family cook, lunch-maker and taxi, dedicated to giving all of my time and energy to my wife and daughters.

CFS had reduced me to a shell of my former self, unable to lift anything heavier than my phone, sometimes not even my own head from the pillow. I was unable to sit at my computer and write a single word for the unrelenting brain fog and cognitive impairment I lived with. I couldn't walk any further than three metres from my bed to the toilet and back. Some days I peed in an empty water bottle beside my bed, as I couldn't get up. My wife washed my hair once a week as I sat on the floor of the shower. My speech became muddled as my tongue lost its ability to wrap itself around words. Sometimes any input of sound amplified my tinnitus and anxiety to the point that I wanted to bang my head against a wall to render myself unconscious. If only I had the energy to do so! I couldn't follow conversations and on many occasions had to tell my daughters to "please just

"I" Was Gone

stop talking", as I couldn't comprehend a word they were saying. I've never felt so useless, crushed and soul-destroyed, knowing I couldn't physically or mentally tolerate listening to one of my daughters simply telling me about her day. I was gone.

AWAKEN WELLNESS

Abandoned in a Broken System

I felt all was lost. I'd been "diagnosed" then abandoned and left to just deal with it. There's a lot to be criticised about how CFS is diagnosed, misdiagnosed, or in some cases completely belittled or ignored by the medical profession. You know there's something wrong in the system when you have to fight to prove the legitimacy of an illness that affects tens of millions worldwide. The standard diagnostic test by elimination is akin to saying "well, we couldn't find anything wrong clinically in your basic blood test, so I'm guessing it's 'x'!" I've been insulted, had general practitioners laugh whilst rolling their eyes at me, some Google-searched for answers in front of me, and I even had one tell me CFS is nothing more than mental illness. There was no knowledge offered, no further clinical testing suggested, no assistance and nothing I could do other than ride it out, which, as I'd been told, could be forever!

This book isn't about doctor-bashing, as many mean well and do amazing things. However, so many are limited, even blinkered in their approach and some have a terrible bedside manner, completely ignorant to the weight their words have on a patient's outlook. Because of their qualifications, people believe they have the answer and for many, it becomes the only answer. And this is where one remains stuck.

Frustration turned to despair as I drowned for a year in the inadequacies of the health system. Lost and fending for myself with barely the cognitive function to read or see, I began the task of searching for answers knowing it was all up to me. I hold no grudges against the individuals who made me feel like a hypochondriac suffering from some kind of undiagnosed mental illness, only disillusionment and confusion that people living with the lowest quality of life are still ignored and dismissed like this by so many health professionals around the world. The medical profession and the methods by which care is delivered and funded should come to terms with the extreme limitations of those afflicted with CFS. People suffering from CFS should not be forced in silence to adapt to the limitations of the health system.

I'd been essentially discarded and left in limbo by the very people and system entrusted with providing answers. I knew nothing about CFS nor had I ever heard of or known anyone else with the condition. I soon discovered hundreds of thousands of fellow Australians are diagnosed CFS sufferers, and many have faced the same disparagement and mistreatment, left to fend for themselves with no offers for further clinical exploration, holistic treatment options or alternatives other than pain management pharmaceuticals and anti-depressants. It is a broken system fuelled by both ignorance and arrogance, and one where treatment is still based on a "one symptom=one drug cure" disease-mongering mentality, mandated by pharmaceutical companies which control not only clinical practices, but also government policy. Healthcare will never improve until patients get involved with fixing it.

People living with chronic illness are often just looking for quality of life advice, and for the most part, many doctors fail miserably in this regard. Instead of providing hopeful advice to CFS sufferers, most respond with a clueless diagnosis and subsequent trial and error medication protocols, instead of really listening and taking into account that they are sitting in a room with an *individual*, with individual symptoms and individual needs requiring an individual plan to test, diagnose and manage to improve their daily life. But there's no time for this. It's much easier to write a prescription and send people on their merry way. Take a number—*next!*

Lack of empathy and patient understanding is a plague amongst many general practitioners who are more interested in watching the clock than taking the time to properly assess one's needs. If more doctors were simply equipped to ask, listen and advise rather than assume, judge and prescribe, more chronic illness sufferers would get the tests and treatment plans they deserve. God forbid you exceed the allotted 10 minutes you're entitled to for your $75.

As a chronic "invisible illness" sufferer, sitting in a room chatting and smiling with a doctor for 10 minutes probably gives them the surface level impression that you're ok. How many of us have had someone say "but you look fine"? What they don't realise is the days of rest you required to build adequate energy to get out of the house, endure a car ride, the hour-long waiting room wait, then the 10 minute appointment where you probably talked for longer than you have in a week. Nor do they understand the impending crash in the days to follow because you broke your routine and encountered more stressful energy than you have in a month. Coping with CFS symptoms from day to day means you learn to adjust to living with high levels of pain and cognitive dysfunction that would seem unimaginable to the healthy person. It becomes your new normal because you simply have no other choice. It is only through education that doctors will begin to understand what CFS is and how devastatingly it removes every part of your normal life. It is only through seeking functional, holistic and dare I say, "alternative" means of treatment will you begin to heal yourself from CFS.

The Thriving Sickness Business

Have you ever thought it strange that traditional medicine is either disregarded or ridiculed by government policy, medical professionals and the ignorant populace, when all Western medicine has been derived from traditional practices only over the past 100 years? The Chinese got it right 10,000 years ago and Western Medicine is trying to catch up when it comes to truly healing the body.

For the invisible illness sufferer, Western Medical treatment comes in organ-destroying chemically packaged form, designed to addict you, the "customer", and mask what's not been dealt with underneath. Pharmaceuticals heal nothing holistically and you are deceiving yourself if you believe CFS will one day vanish by taking a magic pill. Traditional medicine, functional medicine and holistic healing is the way forward to recovery, especially when so many medical professionals either don't understand or won't acknowledge CFS.

Should you find yourself in the unfortunate position of having to try and prove your illness to an arrogant and doubtful doctor, seek help elsewhere. It is easy for me to recommend a naturopath or another holistic practitioner who would probably set you on the path to recovery faster and more safely than an allopathic professional. However, doctors are needed for testing and benefits referral forms, and they know most of us are visiting them seeking an immediate solution, as we have been conditioned

The Thriving Sickness Business

throughout our lives to behave and think as such. Feel sick? See a doctor who will give you something for it!

This attitude and approach to healthcare has spread globally like a plague since a couple of US billionaires took control of medical education in the 1920's. Andrew Carnegie and J.D. Rockefeller saw the emerging pharmaceutical industry they quickly seized financial jurisdiction of as a potential goldmine and succeeded in having all medical schools in the US who did not exclusively adhere to a pharmaceutical approach to medicine closed down. This model is what medical education has been based on now for almost 100 years. There is and has never been anything healthy about the modern healthcare system. It is just disease management.

If you doubt my criticism of the pharmaceutical industry and its co-dependence on the medical profession, here are some interesting current facts. In the US, there are as many representatives of pharmaceutical companies as there are doctors, all competing to get more and more of their product into the hands of prescribing doctors and you, the customer. Also, congress is dictated to by over 100,000 pharmaceutical lobbyists on behalf of their corporations, who have billions of dollars to influence and determine government policy. In many US states, treatment with pharmaceuticals is enforced by law for certain conditions, with threats of involvement of social services for non-compliance. This is evident in regards to what is now an epidemic of children taking anti-depressants, anti-psychotics and other stimulants to treat labels such as ADHD. Six *billion* prescriptions are filled annually in the US! It is a thriving sickness business to the benefit of shareholders and CEO's. The doctors have become company product distributors and the uneducated patients are merely pawns in the game.

I hope everyone who reads this book petitions their country's medical bodies, and governments to formally recognise the value in holistic healing and not supress "alternatives" through policy, as is the case in Australia with the very public ridiculing of energy healing modalities through media advertising and the axing of benefits to such modalities by private health insurance companies. I reiterate my opinions based on experiences so you or those you are caring for aren't met with the same injustice, and if you are, then you are empowered with knowledge to move forward in your journey into seeking answers and recovering. Something has to change, though. We need a patient revolution.

The University of Google

The University of Google

Truly healing from CFS is up to you, and it was like a slap in my pasty, neuralgia-addled face when I came to this realisation myself. Faced with this reality that any chance of healing was all up to me, I knew I had to make a choice. Either give up, or accept my current situation as impermanent and persevere with the belief that I could overcome this. I knew deep within there had to be another way through this hell. I was determined not to live this forever. There had to be more answers other than the lack of, or misinformation I was being fed by medical opinion. I vowed to spend any fortunate minutes of energy or slightly clearer mind to researching my way out of this debilitating and life-destroying condition.

I became a student of the University of Google!

"The University of Google"—this was a term of belittlement, an insult bestowed upon me by an arrogant and narrow-minded upcoming medical student who felt the need to publicly disparage me for showing an active and critical interest in my own health concerns and for expressing the general ignorance toward holistic approaches in treating illness. I was to blindly accept the opinion of this esteemed person because they'd completed a couple of years more tertiary study than myself. I took this slight and used it as fuel for my fire. I was thankful for such a conceited assessment of my intelligence, as it motivated me to be unwavering in my quest to expand my knowledge in every field, and yes, the University of Google was my platform! I'd resolved that

I was on a mission to heal my life and help others, and I would use any source necessary to find the information I needed, not just the limited recommended texts I'm instructed by someone else to read.

It is this blinkered approach still fostered in student learning environments by those supposedly leading the healers of the future that limit mindsets and stifle holistic approaches to health and well being. In our lifetime, we literally have access to the most amount of educational, insightful and consciousness expanding information and research in the history of the world, yet there are those who seek to deride investigators of truth and knowledge like myself for their own egos and interests. I may not have a medical degree on the wall of my office, but I have the world at my fingertips, many years of formal and informal study and practice in varying health, educational, nutritional and healing modalities, and a compulsive urge to never rest on my laurels and never stop learning. I don't need to become a doctor with a superiority complex to help and educate others.

The world is in your hands. There is no ONE way to "cure" CFS, as it is so complex a condition and affects every sufferer uniquely. For this reason, you must dismiss those who try to disparage your journey into self-healing and relentlessly find the answers you seek to achieve any level of improvement you can. Had I listened to this person or relied solely on medical opinion, I would *still* be suffering in bed 22 hours a day waiting for that elusive miracle solution to be handed to me in a pill sometime in the next 5-10-15-20 years.

CFS Schools of Thought

Throughout my University of Google education, I was able to research all of the variables pertaining to CFS. After about a year and a lot of digging, I was also able to find an amazing functional medicine doctor who, along with everything else I was applying to heal myself, was able to educate and set me on the next path to recovery. There are some great specialists in the world who are interested in helping CFS sufferers. It is a damaging summary of the profession however, that these are rare and hard to find, especially to some people who are barely able to read, let alone research where to find an effective CFS literate general practitioner. Every general practitioner should be CFS literate!

To give you an indication of the complexity of the illness and the areas that some dedicated researchers are exploring, I have listed *just some* of the theories, potential causes and treatment possibilities:

- Sluggish brain blood circulation
- Detox
- Hypothalamus-Pituitary-Adrenal axis malfunction
- Mitochondrial dysfunction
- Gluten-free diet
- Paleo diet
- Acupuncture treating Yin deficiency
- Osteopathy and lymphatic drainage
- Oral systemic balance

AWAKEN WELLNESS

- Pyroluria
- Cognitive behavioural therapy
- Natural Killer cell dysfunction
- The Leptin Diet
- Graded exercise therapy
- Mickel Therapy
- Oil Pulling
- Lightning Process
- Gut microbiome changes
- Emotional Freedom Technique
- Adrenal fatigue
- Viral vagus nerve infection
- Negative/ low thyroid TH3 output
- Reverse Therapy
- Leaky gut syndrome
- XMRV
- DHEA
- Long term anti-viral drugs
- Bioidentical cortisol
- Thyroxine
- Far infra red saunas
- Lyme disease
- Autoimmune diseases
- Naturopathy
- Enzyme deactivation
- Epstein Barr Virus
- HHV6
- Low dose Naltrexone
- Traditional Chinese Medicine
- Herbal supplements
- B12 injections
- IV Vitamin C therapy
- Colonics
- AMPK deactivation

CFS Schools of Thought

- Faecal implants
- MTHFR
- Cytokine abnormalities
- Ketogenic Diet
- Craniosacral Therapy
- Intracellular immune dysfunction
- the list goes on and on and on…

I asked my wife to buy me the biggest notebook she could find on her way home one day. My intention was to research everything I could find, compile notes, attempt every possible avenue of healing and track the results. Even when I couldn't write for more than a few minutes (you should see some of my handwriting and spelling on certain days!), I recorded with diligence every single day my diet, activity, energy levels, symptoms, supplements, emotions, sleep patterns, insights and experiences with medical practitioners.

Here is an entry from 2013:

Daily protocol to beat this thing—
Diet: go gluten-free, dairy-free, lots of protein and good fats, juice organic veggies
Exercise: try and walk, stretch
Supplements: learn and regiment
Thinking: stress reduction, coping techniques, gratitude, EFT
Work: healing is your job now, research, focus on goals
Social contact: text, call, Facebook people
Meditation: daily, healing visualisation
CFS workbook: track everything
Pre-emptive rest: stay within the "energy envelope"
Happy activities: ocean, pat the dog, make raw energy snacks, iTunes courses

This became my starting point after some time flailing in

helplessness. There were weeks where I couldn't read, write, walk or talk. But every moment where I was able, I turned to this plan and followed it, determined I would educate my way free from CFS! I implemented this plan after quickly learning of the complex nature of CFS. Some of the aforementioned theories may work for some and not others. Some are pioneering research into causes to try and find treatment options and some are just theories. The fact is, all are acting in isolation from one another and CFS does not act in isolation. There is no single medically documented cause and no one set of symptoms. Therefore, I knew only a whole body holistic and integrative approach to addressing the condition would result in any level of recovery.

Healing from CFS lies in uncovering the systemic failure unique to your brain, body and emotions and transforming every element of them from the inside out with diligence and a daily practice of small, compounding actions toward improvement. You may be as lost as I was at the beginning of my illness, but if you use this book to write your own prescription and determine your own formula for recovery, you will navigate your way through this hell.

The Roadblocks

After a little bit of "why me?" time, I resolved with the deepest of conviction that I would find an answer and heal myself from the seemingly incurable. It is said that acceptance plays a large role in coming to terms with a CFS diagnosis and living with it. The only thing I was going to accept was that I would recover from this temporary setback. With every spare moment of clear-headedness I was briefly blessed with, I was on my computer reading research papers. I became well enough versed to thoroughly understand things that should have been explained to me and tested for from the first instance I presented to a doctor.

Thankfully, my years prior in an incredibly monotonous medical university librarian position afforded me ample time to study medical journals, in between daydreaming and staring out my window at the ocean view! There were times I quite seriously entertained the notion of formally studying to become a doctor, to live up to my namesake and not-too-distant relative, the renowned Professor John Murtagh. However, I've always been interested in far too many things to ever commit to one career. That said, I absorb whatever knowledge I immerse myself in like a sponge and learnt a great deal studying like a medical student whilst a poorly paid librarian! My list of medical experiences informed me, though, that I would have made a far more compassionate and open-minded doctor than most I've encountered.

I was lucky enough to initially find a general practitioner who, whilst not helpful of her own accord, would entertain my research and refer me for any tests I requested. It seemed ridiculous I was telling a doctor how to assess what might be causing symptoms, but I was learning more each month, and she was obliging. Getting this doctor to print a form was easy; actually obtaining results in Australia from competent testing facilities proved near impossible.

Recovering from CFS in a clueless health system that for the most part denies the existence of the illness is challenging to say the least! Should one be struck down with this condition as a resident of the US or UK, there is a plethora of laboratories, testing facilities, treatment clinics and knowledgeable and enthusiastic research specialists at your disposal. Then again, why are so many people suffering in silence in those countries if this is the case? For some reason, Australia seems to be in the dark when it comes to almost all of the above, one exception being a university study passionately dedicated to researching immune biomarkers.

When you barely have the energy to make a phone call or send an email, having the added stress of chasing up results that should have been provided months prior or having 5 vials of blood drawn only then be told a month later, "we don't actually have the resources to do that test here in Australia" is both frustrating and disheartening.

One laboratory in Melbourne lost my adrenal saliva tests. In the meantime, I withered away for months, waiting for an answer in between many infuriating "on-hold" phone sessions that would sap my cognitive energy for weeks after. A pathology collection centre twice took and discarded my bloods for tests that cannot be conducted in Australia. On a separate occasion, I signed up for a university CFS study with the promise of

The Roadblocks

a treatment centre opening soon. I gave 10 vials of blood, after which I experienced a decline in function that lasted for months. I later learned CFS sufferers already have low blood volume as a common trait, and anyone getting even a basic blood test should prepare with electrolytes before and after.

I urge you to empower yourself with knowledge. Take where I've been, and use the lessons I've had to learn on this arduous road to make yours easier. Find a way to get the tests listed in this book, and if your doctor won't oblige, find another who will. It is essential if you're in the early stages of CFS to find a doctor who will do the basic necessary tests immediately to rule out easily treatable underlying conditions, as statistics have proven early intervention greatly improve your chances of recovery.

AWAKEN WELLNESS

Patients: The New Authority

I have put off writing this book for two reasons. The first being that until about a year ago I didn't think I could write anymore. I had barely been able to structure a sentence during my illness until this point, so I had zero confidence in my abilities. Secondly, there is a real fear I experienced as being one to speak out. Being so devastatingly ill long term with CFS can cause some within the community to be despondent and highly critical of anyone who dares to announce they've recovered, let alone try and publicly explain how. I've personally experienced this online where sometimes bitterness reigns over open-minded discussion of theories and ideas.

I've encountered some people like that on my journey, and I truly have compassion for them all, as I know how hard it is to live this way for so long. The fact is, we are all horribly ill when suffering through a life with chronic illness and everyone is ill in different ways, with varying symptoms and levels of dysfunction. We all live with loss. However, it's not a competition for who is the sickest! I once had a stranger remark to me online, "you're lucky to just have CFS! I wish I *just* had CFS," because she suffered from additional conditions. I didn't "just have CFS", but I responded with compassion for her circumstances and explained she had no idea what I encounter day-to-day.

There will be detractors who read this and assume that because I've recovered from CFS that I didn't have "true" CFS or ME, or maybe I *just* had adrenal fatigue or maybe I'm *just* tired.

Patients: The New Authority

There will probably even be detractors who don't read this book at all, but will criticise its very existence because I'm offering self-healing pathways to the seemingly incurable. Because of the level of suffering experienced by people, it seems anyone who pops their head up having recovered and offering hope or alternatives to waiting for that elusive allopathic cure is often ridiculed and shot down. I risk that. I risk being derided by both the sick and the medical profession for my assessment of the system and my relaying of experiences. Also, I'm not a doctor and this isn't a research paper. It is the result of years of desperation and application, scribbling notes, researching from any and every random medical source I could find when I could barely read or write. I may be somewhat of a layperson, but I have done more research into CFS than any general practitioner I encountered over the years, and have found what worked for me. I was forced to become my own authority on the subject and you will find you must also. When faced with the barrage of symptoms combined with the medical ignorance I was faced with as a CFS sufferer, self-study is the only study!

People should respect one another going through this. It will be more helpful for people to implement every strategy herein that will lead to cumulative improvement of any level, rather than waiting for researchers in a lab somewhere to hand them the magical solution. We all wait in suffering if we rely on such a solution. We face symptoms that no normal human could possibly tolerate every minute of every day, and we face it over and over again, some of us for decades. It doesn't have to be this way, though.

Admittedly there are some charlatans who feel the need to cash in on the sick by offering false hope. I have experienced some in all of my trials, and I'm sure you have too. But I own my story; my story is my credential, and I'm sharing my truth as I have lived it to help as many people as I can. As you will learn from my experience, recovering from CFS isn't just eating whole grains and exercising! CFS is a complete systemic biological, emotional and spiritual breakdown of astronomical proportions, and every facet of this must be addressed and rebuilt for any hope of recovery. Having the least amount of energy and being hit with the most complex devastating array of symptoms you'll ever have in your life, then having to do the greatest amount of work you'll ever have to do to be well again, seems insurmountable! Yet in a system that has no answers or support and a society ignorant to the reality of living with this illness, this is what CFS sufferers face. I can only offer an insight into my personal experience and I hope it inspires you to take action and start piecing together your own health puzzle.

I know how challenging this will be for you. I know how insufferably poor the quality of life is for CFS sufferers. I've lived it. The misery is ongoing and has been documented to be a lower quality of life than someone with renal failure or heart disease. If we had cancer we would then at least get recognition from the medical community! I've had people tell me there's always someone worse off, and it's an insult to what you have to live with day to day, as I'm sure you'll agree. I would never diminish the seriousness of a life with CFS, nor compare my journey to that of another.

But if you feel resentful because you are so ill, let it go. There are warriors everywhere facing battles with cancer, lupus, MS, mental illness, endometriosis, cerebral palsy, muscular dystrophy (the list goes on), that you know little about. If you encounter

Patients: The New Authority

someone who is recovering and healing from any chronic illness, congratulate and communicate with them. They've probably worked their butt off at every level of their mind, body and spirit to gain even the slightest improvement, like I have, and there is probably something to learn from them. Release the bitterness and cynicism, as it only harms your system and also brings down the person who is improving. I've seen too many elated CFS sufferers immediately deflated by the mob online because they're healing themselves.

Everyone can tap into the tenacity within to begin to understand and heal from CFS. It will require that you own your personal journey, become your own authority, and try everything you believe will help you as an individual. You should be open to healing yourself on every level using every possible resource, instead of following the doctor's advice to "take some pain meds and stay home in bed," as I was repeatedly told. Recovering from CFS is not about fighting others, resistance or comparison, but gaining an understanding of nurturing your whole self, developing self-compassion and dissolving stress and emotional upheaval. If you can channel your energy into mastering these aspects of yourself, you will be on your way to healing.

AWAKEN WELLNESS

To the Healthy Person

This book is for well people too. It's for super healthy vibrant people who have never been struck down by illness. It's for these fortunate people too, so they may gain an awareness of the plight of those struggling in silence every second of every day with chronic illness. I hope they learn something from my story about the loss, the battle, the pain and hardship I endured, for it is not in isolation. Millions around the world lay in darkened rooms, living with pain and torment a fully healthy person will never be able to understand. I hope to give a voice to these people, because not too long ago, this was me. I hope people are inspired by my story enough to go out into the world and share it, help someone in need or even begin to raise awareness within their circle or community about the interconnectedness of physical and emotional health and wellness.

I hope people are woken up by my experience with and assessment of the broken healthcare system, and are motivated to shake it up and change it in ways that benefit those who truly need care and assistance. Those who can barely lift their head from a pillow aren't the ones capable of instigating the changes that need to happen. It is up to me. And it is with encouragement I offer the challenge to you as well.

In February 2013, there was a young woman in Denmark named Karina Hansen who, at 23, was taken from her home by psychiatrists, social workers and police against her will and placed in a psychiatric institution. This happened despite clinical evidence of her never having any mental health issues, but rather because she had been diagnosed with chronic fatigue syndrome. The Danish authorities don't believe CFS to be an actual illness, and people who suffer from it are routinely subjected to this kind of abduction there and in some other European countries, and forced into institutions with no family access allowed. Karina's doctors have been denied access to her and her family's attorney has not been provided with any legal documentation to evaluate the lawfulness of her incarceration. Whatever "treatment" Karina has been subjected to by psychiatrists whilst locked away, she now has clinical brain damage.

Never judge someone with an invisible illness. It is not depression, nor is it all in their heads. It's depressing having everything you wanted to do with your life removed by chronic illness. The world needs more compassion and less judgement. Anyone can be struck down with CFS. I have read stories written by doctors, athletes and famous people who have all had their lives turned upside down by CFS. No one is immune. I was very fit, active, intelligent and pursuing various interests when CFS hit me. I now have a few lingering cognitive difficulties and endurance issues since recovering, but my mind is stronger and my body cleaner than it has even been, and I will use every day of my newfound life to make a difference.

Every day is an opportunity to make a difference, both within yourself and to your community and world around you. There are no boundaries anymore in this world. You could start a crowd funding campaign right now to raise funds for CFS research, chronic illness sufferers who can't pay the bills, or even start a social media campaign to petition your government to change funding and treatment models for chronic illnesses like CFS.

Anything is possible, and the help the world needs is limited only by your willingness and drive to make a difference, or your level of apathy to be content in allowing someone like Karina Hansen to vanish into the shadows of a broken and self-serving medical system.

Become Your Own Guinea Pig

Whilst I'm critical of our broken health system when it comes to diagnosing and treating CFS and its associated conditions, please don't despair. The world's information is literally at your fingertips. Study after study is released worldwide almost weekly from dedicated international researchers. There can be some information overload once you start digging, but the nature of CFS is so complex, so challenging and so unique for every sufferer, that it is necessary to find the combination to YOUR puzzle pieces in order to heal.

During my illness, I met a biochemist-turned-naturopath who had, himself, recovered from CFS. At that point in time I was getting frustrated, as I felt like I was doing everything right, yet had plateaued – I was somewhat functional but still crashing. His words resonated with my achiever personality type when he said, "you're doing everything right except for being patient." It's a blasé statement to make, because the loss of living with CFS is devastating. However, it is true in its simplicity. Do everything right and have patience knowing every day you are rebuilding and recovering.

I hope some of the contents of this book make your journey easier. I also hope to enlighten you as to information and modalities you may not have yet considered exploring to recover. I hope you are inspired to never give up, to persist and find that inner strength and conviction to gradually put into practice everything I have learnt to heal yourself from CFS. All of the information contained within helped me transform from a bed-ridden shell of a human who was told to just live this way forever, to someone who recently flew overseas and walked 21 kilometres in 48 hours in New Zealand!

The Broken Body

The Broken Body

I have always been an active person. I love mountain bike riding and used to race downhill as fast as I could over the side of the Great Dividing Range. I have played drums since I was 13 years old and played a lot of amazing live shows in my 20s and 30s, recorded albums and worked as a session musician with some talented players. Playing drums in a hardcore metal band is a physical workout like no other! I have studied different martial arts and self-defence systems over the years, including Krav Maga and Tai Chi, and have always been interested in energy flow in the body. I have always loved the ocean, swimming and surfing as well as long walks along the beach. Bushwalking and hiking also feeds my soul. Before getting ill, I'd jumped on the Crossfit craze, and was physically punishing my body in a way I'd never experienced with high repetition heavy weights workouts. But I was becoming fitter than I'd ever been, so I thought it was all worth it.

That said, I was highly addicted to sugar and caffeine. It was normal for me to eat two Snickers bars, a block of chocolate or a packet of Tim Tams every night. Come 8:30pm was "the chocolating hour!" I cooked healthy meals for my family, but they were almost always pasta based, such was our love of Italian foods and my love of cooking them. I ate pies, donuts and chocolate whenever I felt like it, as I thought it was ok given all the strenuous physical activity I was "balancing" my life with. Strong black espresso coffees fuelled my days and nights and it was nothing

The Broken Body

for me to research and bang out a high distinction level 5000 word university essay the night before it was due.

Despite being a sugar-gorging idiot, my interest in nutritional studies was piqued around the time I began getting strange health issues that didn't seem to disappear. Like the usual non-medically qualified member of society, I'd visit the doctor expecting a solution when the entire time the solution was both controllable and researchable by me. Most general practitioners prescribe pharmaceuticals to attempt to counter whatever symptoms you present them with. That's it. But as Hippocrates said "let food be thy medicine and medicine be thy food." My personal experiences with the profession proved general practitioners have forgotten this. The mantra "first, do no harm," is cast aside too, given the carelessness and ease with which dangerous pharmaceuticals are prescribed.

Let me give you a couple of personal examples. New years day 2010 I woke up with an awful bladder pain. I'd never experienced such a thing before. It didn't subside after Ibuprofen so I visited a doctor who, despite the urine analysis indicating no infection, prescribed antibiotics. I took these for two weeks and still the bladder inflammation persisted. By this stage it had become unbearable, so I was sent for a bladder ultrasound in the Emergency Department, which indicated nothing untoward, and I was referred to a urologist. It was a one-year wait in the public system, and a two-month wait to pay a private physician. I opted to pay a private specialist, but in the meantime, I turned to medical journals to research possible causes and solutions. In my studies, I kept coming back to the term "interstitial cystitis", as all of my symptoms indicated the condition, so I basically diagnosed myself with it in order to begin nutritionally treating it! I put myself on a strict "IT" diet, giving up all acid-causing inflammatory foods. Gone were my beloved coffees and chocolate, as were tomato products and white foods like pasta and breads. The difference was phenomenal and by the time I had my urologist appointment I felt it was almost a waste of time and money going. I had also studied the treatments urologists were likely to use to "heal" conditions like IT, prostatitis and bladder inflammation. Most common was the use of the fluoroquinolone class of antibiotics like Ciprofloxacin. "Cipro" has been widely reported to cause psychiatric disturbances and in many cases, a rupturing of the Achilles tendons!

Readied with this knowledge, I attended my appointment I'd waited two months for (thankfully not in pain, because of the success of my own nutritional research and self-treatment). Within 10 minutes of relaying my symptoms, I had a script for "Cipro" in my hand that I didn't want. I asked if there were any other options and was met with a shrug: "Well, I could probably have a look with a cystoscope, but that'd cost you about a grand." I mentioned I physically trained a lot and if there were any side effects worth noting from this drug and received the response (i.e. lie) "nothing major." I was $330 out of pocket from the healing prowess of this smug medical professional! From that day I learned not to blindly trust another just because of the extra letters after their name, but rather their character and knowledge and mutual reciprocation of ideas and theories. Nothing is ever black and white, and I think, as a CFS sufferer, you know this all too well yourself.

It was with this mentality I faced my next dubious medical encounter. A year later I'd begun to experience a strange facial numbness and migraines. I was initially diagnosed with a

The Broken Body

condition called Bell's Palsy, despite having no obvious facial drop or paralysis, which is the main symptom of the condition. This numbness persisted for months, and I was eventually referred to a neurologist who suggested I have an MRI scan of my brain to rule out Multiple Sclerosis. It was a scary wait thinking that MS was a possibility. In the mean time I'd learnt about the use of magnesium and B12 in treating hemiplegic migraines, another term the neurologist initially used as a possible diagnosis. During my follow up appointment with the neurologist, I mentioned this and he replied (and I'm not even joking), "What are you talking about that for? The body doesn't even *need* minerals." I was dumbfounded! His cure for my migraines and facial numbness was to prescribe me the anti-depressant Endep and a heart medication for high blood pressure (which I've never had) called Lopressor. I refused to start taking either. Again, from two neurologist appointments and a full fee MRI scan, I was out of pocket around $2500. Thankfully I didn't have MS, but I had a lifetime of physiology destroying pharmaceutics my body didn't need at the ready!

It was two weeks later when I visited my chiropractor, still experiencing the same symptoms. Using Kinesiology testing methods, he put his finger on a tooth and said, "get this checked right away." The following day a dental x-ray confirmed a massive abscess above what I thought was a good tooth and I was told this might be causing my symptoms from pressure on the cranial nerve. I had a root canal and a month after this was completed I was entirely free from all facial numbness and migraines.

I have gained more healing from chiropractic, acupuncture and nutritional medicine than from the advice or pharmaceutical recommendations of any medical professional. I acknowledge many specialists have an important place and do help a lot of people, especially in emergency and trauma situations. Not to mention the tireless dedication to healing and caring those in the Nursing profession display. When you're in a hospital bed, a kind word from a caring nurse will beat any painkiller. But from personal experience, I know the concept of functional medicine and holistic healing doesn't even appear on the radars of Western Medicine. That fraternity would rather stick a Band-Aid over a festering wound so when you present again in six months time, they can stick a bigger, more expensive Band-Aid over the same wound.

Healing your body is possible, but it is up to you. You have everything within to do so. It is essential you become an investigator of your self to try and trace your symptoms to a root cause. This will take some effort, honesty and soul searching as well as a lot of discipline and intestinal fortitude in application, but what have you got to lose? I had nothing left in me when I realised this was the choice I had to make to heal my life. You can lead yourself, not only to self-healing, but a life of flourishing beyond what you could have hoped for. You just have to do the work. All of this information is just information. It is when you decide to apply this information you will see change and transformation.

Start now.

Know Your Past, Heal Your Future

Something I believe is essential in beginning to piece together your puzzle is going back in time and writing down all possible contributors to your body not currently functioning in an optimal state. These may be poor dietary habits, stressful events, chemical exposures and illnesses. Awareness of these events when you begin to educate yourself about your condition often leads to light-bulb moments that can take you down a treatment path which will be effective for you. Even though it feels like CFS comes "from nowhere", it definitely came from somewhere, and you already know the answer. You just need to find it.

For me it was a number of physiological and stressful contributing descent factors that all gradually weakened my entire system until that final viral result briefly destroyed my life:

- I have always been a highly anxious person with a poor emotional response to stress, causing my adrenals to work overtime for much of my life. I suffered from panic disorder and agoraphobia from 2002-2004.
- For many years I was highly addicted to sugar and caffeine which weakened my gut and adrenals.
- Following a back injury in which I herniated three lumbar discs in 2007, I overused Voltaren (non-steroidal anti-inflammatory drugs or NSAIDS) so I could keep working pain-free, causing me to develop duodenitis.
- I was placed on the drug Somac for two years as a result of this gut inflammation and later learnt Somac inhibits the

body's ability to absorb B12 and Magnesium by destroying gut integrity.
- For three months in 2010 I unknowingly drank from an installed contaminated water filter in our new house causing me an extended period of gastro-intestinal illness.
- In 2011 I experienced mystery weakness, face numbness and migraines for six months and eventually had a root canal for an abscess above what I thought was a healthy tooth. I now also question the efficacy of root canal procedures.
- In 2012 we bought a brand new mattress that emitted an unbearable chemical solvent smell for months, during which time I experienced sinusitis.
- For many years I endured a lot of stressful extended family issues I had no control over that greatly affected me emotionally.
- I overtrained physically during this stressful period to try and counter the emotional strain, at times lying on the floor of my garage in a heap urging myself to get up and complete another set of deadlifts. I was dehydrated, stressed, depleted and not absorbing nutrients effectively.
- Throughout this decade, I intermittently suffered from recurring viruses.

Given this list, it probably comes as no surprise I became so ill! CFS can be seen as somewhat of a mystery, though here is a clear combination of ongoing and interconnected physiological, environmental and emotional stress. During this time I saw these events as little setbacks, so I would just keep on going, though getting through every day was a challenge. I was still working, studying, writing, playing music, caring for my daughters and maintaining our home. But I was disconnected from my body for many years, ignoring these signals to listen and change what I was doing to myself with stress, medications, toxic people and bad food. Different (and often multiple) triggers can cause CFS in every individual, and because of that, there is no singular healing pathway that will work for everyone. It is an individualised process, just as the condition is unique in each person. This is where the "think happy thoughts and exercise" school of healing CFS fails sufferers. CFS was the worst signal to change I could have ever asked for, but the recovery process improved every aspect of my being in ways I will clarify.

The Virus Myth– Which Came First?

Almost everyone who suffers from CFS can pinpoint that *moment* or event that immediately triggered the condition. Some recount a flu they never recovered from or a traumatic event that instantly sent them down the spiral. For myself, it was like an instantaneous virus of epic proportions knocked me on my arse where I stayed in the acute stage for well over a year. Research is now pointing to evidence there is actually a lot going on in the body before this "trigger" and we just fail to notice until it's too late. Preceding CFS, the immune system is overworking in the background often for many years due to physical, emotional or environmental stress. Stress coping mechanisms remain on high alert and operating at this level becomes normal to you. Your body is a very resilient instrument but eventually it reaches a point where it can't take any more.

Chronic hyperactivity of the sympathetic nervous system through emotional or environmental strain triggers the hypothalamus to go into and remain stuck in high-alert mode. This will then instigate the immune system to produce far too many T-cells and cytokines, causing the body to essentially fight itself in response to what is perceives as a threat. Viral symptoms ensue, and the immune system works even harder to recover before more opportunistic viral symptoms appear and eventually don't seem to go away. Endocrine disruption supervenes, and hormonal imbalances follow before that final trigger sends your body into what becomes CFS. A virus does not *cause* CFS, it is merely, for many, the final straw and an end result. A virus is in fact an *effect*, not a cause.

Speaking personally, I had undergone a lot of self-inflicted physical stress and endured my share of emotional stress in the years leading up to succumbing to CFS. Given all of the elements in your life you're then tasked with healing, it's no wonder CFS can be seen for some as a massive wake up call. It definitely was for me! So there may well be an immune biomarker, a persistent underlying infection, or a history of gut dysfunction, but the initial hypothalamic disruption that precedes all of these factors is where the answer lies. With this in mind, it can be proposed this condition is helping alert you to changes you need to make in your life. You have lived at a malfunctioning level for far too long and your body is trying to tell you enough is enough. There is always a reason in addition to and beyond the physical symptoms that have to be dealt with, and when these reasons are addressed, your body will regain homeostasis.

Healing the Broken Body

Healing the body from CFS requires a total transformation of every aspect of yourself. Forget who you were. What got you into this is not what will get you out of this. By that, I mean you have to become a whole new person (or a new *whole* person) to completely overcome this incapacitating condition. You must work in small progressive steps every single day on changing your diet, stress response, how you breathe, what you do, what gives you joy, letting go of limiting beliefs and old patterns of thinking that no longer serve you, becoming educated about your body, nutrition, supplements, environmental chemicals and toxins, becoming aware of the agriculture industry and what is happening to the foods we eat, the household products and cosmetics used every day, and eliminating the toxic people from your life who drain you emotionally. You have to think bigger than the present conditions in your life for anything to change.

You must become a master of your destiny, not a victim of your history. YOU have to do this! It takes effort and discipline but you have to do it all to piece your physiology and stress response back together and eliminate unhealthy things from your life permanently in every form. You can't try one thing for a little while and then give up because it didn't work. You have to do all things, all the time! There wouldn't be a CFS sufferer alive who doesn't want to recover and live a life of health and vitality. You know this is what you want. So you must ask yourself every day: *what can I do today that will bring me closer to what I want?*

Healing the Broken Body

The answers lay within and this guide for your healing journey will teach you how to restore a physical body that is essentially malfunctioning.

If you are undertaking any kind of healing protocol, whether you are newly affected by CFS or have suffered for many years, it is essential you establish your baseline capabilities first, heal your gut so nutrients can begin to be effectively absorbed once you introduce supplements, rectify your sleeping patterns and then begin to address mitochondrial dysfunction and testing for hormonal issues. Throughout this time, it will be vital to begin to build your emotional resources, so feel free at any stage to turn to the relevant sections of this book for tools to empower you as you progress.

Enjoying Pacing

Pacing can be both a limiting word and a cause of even more stress in CFS patients. Too much emphasis has been placed on pacing and graded exercise therapy as the cure or the way to manage CFS forever. In the early stages of CFS it is indeed necessary to realise your body's limits and pace yourself, as you are trapped in a depleted system that is just keeping your vital organs running. Stressing your mitochondria so it can't keep up with demand will cause a painful crash through the build up of lactic acid that occurs once your body slips into anaerobic metabolism to cope with such strain. It helps to determine first of all what your baseline level of activity is. This is the level you are comfortable doing something at, so as not to exacerbate your pain symptoms in the early acute stages of your illness.

It is often referred to as "staying within the energy envelope", and is a far more clinically sensible way of managing CFS than graded exercise therapy will ever be. The resting lactate levels of a CFS sufferer (clinically proven by muscle biopsy) are as high as those found in marathon runners. High lactate levels are attributed to the body's complete breakdown of aerobic energy production, relying on anaerobic energy production and the consequent flood of chemicals that collect causing pain. Graded exercise therapy does not help a physical system trapped in this state, but you will learn to implement more effective strategies that can and will undo this chemical overload.

When I was in the worst of it, my baseline/marathon was

Enjoying Pacing

walking to the kitchen and back to my bedroom. Because of this fact, I had to consider what I needed to complete in the harrowing 15 metre return journey! I should get a drink, some food and go to the toilet within this trip, as I may not be able to move to make another one for the next 6 hours. That was my reality on a "good day" for a very long time.

Your baseline may be showering, hanging up the washing or walking the dog for 10 minutes without causing post-exertional fatigue and pain. Whatever it is, establish that and then gradually try to increase through *enjoyable* experiences rather than chores or targets. Once I was able to walk up the street 100 metres, I worked hard on pushing and pushing until I could walk around the block for 5 minutes, trying to implement graded exercise therapy, as I was lead to believe it would help me to recover quickly. I would then crash hard not knowing why. I figured out I wasn't enjoying the self-imposed increase in monotonous activity, was stressing about the whole process and my body was shutting me down again as a result. Graded exercise therapy is like forcing yourself to run with torn ligaments that haven't yet healed. You can only cause more damage to a body not yet able to cope with exercise-by-obligation as therapy. I spent rest time in states of horizontal worry stressing about my exercise limitations, rather than allowing myself to be in a healing mindset.

In this sense, pacing as a term can be limiting when you are mentally reinforcing your limits on a daily and sometimes hourly basis. Pacing contradicts the concept of pursuing happy and fulfilling experiences, as you're constantly restricting yourself with fear something bad will happen should you get out there and enjoy yourself. I did this to myself for a long time, diligently planning any outing within strict parameters and timeframes, for fear of what might happen should I extend beyond my self-imposed limits. I know all too well the pain that comes with over-exertion, so I'm not suggesting you jump into downhill mountain bike riding and ignore your body, but from my experience with changing limiting beliefs and the impact that can have on physical healing, I recommend your "pacing" becomes a strategy of how to enjoy yourself more at a level that allows you to cope free from the fear your body will "pay you back" for doing so. Developing the mental strategies you will learn throughout this book will stem the chemical reactions causing the symptoms that, for now, won't allow you to move freely.

Take Out the Trash!

A by-product of the modern environment we live in is an accumulative toxic load on our system. If you eat supermarket foods, wear cosmetics and deodorant, breathe city air, take medications and have amalgam fillings, then you have accumulated toxins in your body throughout your life (and this basically means everyone!) There are over 80,000 human-made chemicals that can enter our daily lifestyle. Every one of these toxins that enter our system alters the ways in which our biochemistry works and cells function. They block the ability of the mitochondria to function effectively and also compound as we add to the toxic load within us on a daily basis through our dietary and household choices. However, every human being is different and some are unable to process and clear toxins, and for some the energy pathways become blocked for this reason alone.

Detoxing your system is one of the necessary first steps toward healing your body. Your body will become more receptive to absorbing nutrients from foods and supplements. You will go through a stage of feeling a bit worse, so it is best to proceed slowly and gently. This is scary thought for CFS sufferers and I know it all too well – when you feel as bad as you do, the concept of feeling even worse is a daunting one. However, this brief period is simply a "Herxheimer's Reaction" (a *herx* or healing crisis), whereby the immune system is processing dead organisms faster than your body can expel them. This indicates your body is entering a state of healing. Keep telling yourself this is necessary for your body to heal.

There are a few ways to make this process more manageable and aid detox:

- Starting your day with fresh lemon squeezed in water wakes up your liver and alkalises your digestive system.
- Bragg's Organic Apple Cider Vinegar is also great for alkalising the system.
- Lymphatic drainage can be very helpful in moving toxins along faster through the lymph channels. Definitely avoid any strenuous deep tissue or sports massage.
- Turmeric is great for detoxifying the liver and also increases the body's production of Glutathione, also known as the master antioxidant.
- Infrared saunas have proven benefits, though I never tried these myself.
- Chlorella is helpful for chelating metals and removing them from the system.
- Taking milk thistle prior to commencing any detox will strengthen and tonify your liver.
- Dry skin brushing followed by Epsom salt baths helps release toxins through your largest organ, the skin, and also increases the body's absorption of magnesium.

I will elaborate further on this, but it is essential to eat only organic foods where possible and to avoid a diet of processed foods. This isn't a temporary suggestion; this is from now on, forever. Reduce and eliminate any exposure to mould, which is toxic. Also switching to natural skin care products and making your household as chemical-free as humanly possible will greatly increase your quality of life. It's amazing to know that simple white vinegar can replace almost all the chemical cleaning products in your home!

Who Pulled the Plug?

I have followed the pioneering work of UK fatigue specialist Dr Sarah Myhill from the outset of my journey living with CFS. Dr Myhill uses the analogy of the "engine room" of the body to explain mitochondrial dysfunction and its effects on health. One of the keys to digging free from debilitating fatigue is to address and correct mitochondrial dysfunction. The mitochondria are the engines living in every cell of every living organism and are basically responsible for keeping life going. They take fuel from your body and together with oxygen, produce adenosine triphosphate (ATP) as the fuel for your body.

When ATP is being efficiently recycled in the body you are able to live normally, work and cope with the demands of life. However, when demand exceeds delivery, your body can switch to a dysfunctional state, producing a substance called AMP that takes a long time to drain from your body and recycle into ATP. This explains, to a certain extent, the sense of delayed fatigue following energy expenditure. In this state of extreme depletion you are essentially being protected from over-stressing your heart and organs. If you pushed through them, your body would simply stop living.

So what causes mitochondrial dysfunction?

Life places so may demands on our bodies and we often fail to realise the effect the plethora of environmental toxins, emotional stress and poor nutritional choices has over time. Lack of nutrients and minerals, gut dysfunction and environmental stressors, whether they are emotional or chemical, all affect and block mitochondrial function. When you take into account two-thirds of our total energy expenditure is used by our body simply functioning as it should to keep us alive, there isn't a lot left to expend and even less in an acute CFS sufferer whose body is literally just keeping you alive.

As someone with CFS, I'm sure you know the feeling like you have been unplugged. There is nothing left. Some nights I couldn't even lift my fork to my mouth. Some days I crawled to the toilet and then collapsed and stayed on the floor for a couple of hours to build the energy for the crawl back to bed.

It is imperative you understand the impact every choice you make has on your cellular energy function, so you can begin to correct and restore yourself. By detoxing both physically and emotionally, correcting your gut, fuelling your body with nutritional food and supplements, and uncovering possible sources of infection or hormonal dysfunction, you will begin to restore your mitochondrial function.

Who Pulled the Plug?

Nutrition: Healing the Second Brain

Healing the gut is absolutely crucial as a starting point to recovery from CFS or any chronic illness. The gut is referred to as "the second brain" for the significance with which its level of wellness controls immune function, brain chemistry and most of the biological functions that power and maintain your body. The old adage "you only get out what you put in" could not be more appropriate.

For years, I fuelled myself with chocolate, bread, sugar, caffeine, take-away burgers and donuts and expected to be able to physically train myself at an elite level in my home gym! In reality, I was barely making it through each day. I tolerated inflammatory conditions in my back and knees and tore three of the four rotator cuff tendons in my left shoulder. I rode a rollercoaster of hypoglycaemia and dizziness because of my sugar consumption habits, and rarely had a night of restorative sleep. I was reactive to any external conditions emotionally, frequently angry, as well as slumping into depressive states as my poor dietary choices wreaked havoc with my moods and brain chemistry. I developed duodenitis and gastritis from overusing non-steroidal anti-inflammatory drugs to ironically (i.e. stupidly) try and cope with injury and the inflammation I was bringing upon my body. As a result, I was placed on the drug Somac, a proton pump inhibitor, designed to reduce gastric symptoms. In effect, this drug rid my gut of its ability to produce hydrochloric acid for optimal food digestion, as well as inhibiting my body's ability to absorb nutrients, most notably vitamin B12, needed for a host of neurological and biological functions. And still, at 8:30 every night, I would eat two Snickers bars!

Fast forward to my life post-CFS and I am ashamed of the garbage-disposal I once was. I no longer eat any gluten, dairy, sugar or processed foods. It may sound rather limiting, but I now live on an array of lean meats, chicken, fish, nuts, seeds, organic fruits and vegetables, avocados, berries, rice, healthy oils, eggs, fermented vegetables and hemp protein powder. I cook an assortment of stir-fries, curries made from scratch and variations on protein and veg. Healthy doesn't have to be boring; it just takes some creativity, knowledge and forethought. Have you noticed how many different vegetables exist? I also make a variety of snacks with my food processor so in my mind, I still get "treats"-they're just super-healthy! Throughout my recovery I tried to follow a vegetable intake to boost mitochondrial function that I'd read a Multiple Sclerosis patient was having success with. This included several cups per day of green leafy vegetables, lots of variety in bright colours as well as plenty of omega 3's from grass-fed beef and salmon. I eat roughly every 2.5 hours (five small meals per day) to keep my blood sugar steady and protein with every meal. I now live happily with no pain in my knees, shoulder or back, no pharmaceuticals, no digestive issues, no bloating, steady blood sugar, no dizziness, I'm non-reactive to stress and I have a happy, optimistic disposition.

This section will help you begin to adapt to your limitations in a way that will slowly rebuild your nutritional health. I will briefly outline what helps and what harms and how you can manage with restricted energy levels to consume healthy foods each day. Because of the importance of gut healing and nutrition, I highly recommend you work with a nutritionist to tailor a personal plan to support your recovery.

Gluten: the Inflammatory Monster

One of the first steps I undertook on my pathway to better nutritional health was to eliminate gluten from my diet. I was someone who grew up on sandwiches, pastas and packaged cereals, so this was a challenging transition from feeling I needed to have bread with every meal to eating primarily proteins and salads. The first reason you should give up gluten is because modern wheat is so far removed from the nutritional staple it once was. It is a genetically modified and poisonous non-food. Secondly, gluten-containing foods contain the gliadin molecule that binds to your cells and trigger an immune response in sensitive individuals and those with already stressed systems. That's us! The immune system actually makes antibodies to attack the healthy cells the gliadins have permeated because your body thinks you have an infection. This immune response depletes an already malfunctioning system and compromises your overall chances of healing your body.

After eliminating gluten from my diet I felt slightly worse for a month, but after this time noticed my belly had shrunk, my cravings for anything sweet had gone and my moods had begun to improve. It can take a month for the gut inflammation to subside, and a few more months for the lining of the small intestine to heal completely, but it pays to become disciplined with your nutritional health. Filling your body with allergenic foods keeps your system on high alert by constantly triggering an immune response.

Going Organic vs Eating Glycophosphates

Our agriculture system is now chronically depleted of minerals, compared to the levels that used to exist. Minerals are no longer in the foods at the levels we need to function optimally. Over time, deficiencies are guaranteed and this is where much of the population sits, even when eating well. At the behest of the greed of companies like Monsanto, intent on altering and controlling the world's food supply, almost all "grown" food is now manipulated, altered and toxic. Glycophosphate, the main chemical in the pesticide "Round-Up", infects much of the agriculture worldwide and is devastatingly toxic to the body. The decision to go completely organic is not some new age weirdness you can be dismissive of. It is a necessity to eliminate all pesticide-laden foods and rid these toxins from your organs so your body can begin to heal.

Detoxing from 37 years of pesticide consumption took a while! But the decision to go completely organic is one I'll never regret. People baulk at the slightly higher cost, but what does a life of illness cost? I still eat and juice organic vegetables daily and will forever. A meal to me in the afternoon could simply be a handful of almonds and a carrot. You need to think of the long-term outcome and make wise choices every time you step into the kitchen. It's too easy to reach for poor food choices when, for some of us, it may be the only joy in our days! However, you must realise that every time you open your mouth and fill it with

Gluten: the Inflammatory Monster

a chemical pesticide-laden or processed "food" product, you are giving away your power, your health and adding to the burden your organs and digestive system are already under.

Avoid Processed Sugars

After eliminating gluten, I initially felt a bit limited with what I could and couldn't eat. One of the added bonuses, though, is I stopped eating a lot of packaged foods, and therefore gave up all forms of processed sugar and additives as a result. Sugar and, in particular, the high fructose corn syrup that is becoming prevalent as a cheap alternative sugar in most processed foods, wreaks havoc with your body. The kidney energy is vital in Chinese medicine and a diet with any amount of HFCS destroys this energy, stresses your liver and also leads to insulin resistance and blood pressure issues. A body running on processed sugar and fructose disrupts metabolism, with the liver retaining the toxins and forced to convert most of it to fat. I mentioned I lived on a diet extremely high in processed sugar before my descent into CFS; a diet I thought I could just 'train away.' It's sad some people wait for trauma to decide to change their life, and I was one of them.

Alternatives to sugar that I use in my raw food super-snacks are organic maple syrup and dates. Stevia is fine as a sweetener, though I avoid agave syrup as it has been shown to metabolise and produce an insulin response in the body the same way as HFCS. Once you lose the unhealthy-sweet tooth addiction and bombardment of sugar to your system, your inflammation levels in your body will rapidly subside and your hormonal levels will begin to stabilise as a result. You'll also find fruits are sweet enough. I haven't eaten a chocolate bar, donut or biscuit for years

Avoid Processed Sugars

now and putting food like that in my body isn't something I'll even contemplate risking. I value the progress I've made and the new life I now have too much to become undisciplined and re-poison my body.

Eat Every 2.5 Hours

Another helpful step I undertook was to begin eating 5 meals a day with protein included in every meal. This helps to allay hypoglycaemia and the symptoms of having too much insulin in the blood such as dizziness. Balancing blood sugar levels is the key to not only proper regulation of the circadian rhythm, but also the homeostasis of cortisol adrenal output. That said, I know what it's like to have zero energy and in my early stages of CFS it took all I had within me to get seven metres to the kitchen to fetch myself a snack. Meal preparation when you barely have the energy to move your arms and legs makes it near impossible to follow any kind of eating regime.

However, by having your partner or a family member prepare things in advance for you, or doing so yourself when you have a window of energy, it will be easier to grab-and-go with a healthy choice meal than a microwaved dinner or packaged poison when you are experiencing down days (or weeks). I used to grate organic vegetables (beetroot, carrots, zucchini, kale) into separate containers and refrigerate boiled eggs. That way I had protein and salad meals on hand whenever I needed without stressing about *how* I was going to make something to eat that would nourish my body when I could barely make it to the kitchen. I would simply scoop out a spoonful of each into a bowl – instant salad!

Cortisol and the Gut

Eating with the aforementioned pattern and reducing stress by adapting your meal preparation to align with your current physical state does wonders for depleted adrenal glands and helps them to better regulate cortisol production. You are able to respond more effectively to the stress your body is currently facing if you can ease the workload of your adrenals. I learnt during my quest for nutritional healing the importance of gut health in controlling your immune response.

Cortisol levels determine the immune response in your gut. If you are stressing your body and your adrenals are going haywire, as is the case with all CFS sufferers, the gut immune response suffers and tissues become inflamed and damaged. The body reacts by producing toxins and slowing digestion and blood flow to the intestines. As a result, unhealthy bacteria are free to multiply and thrive, further stressing your immune response. It's a vicious cycle that proliferates, and one of the many ways CFS can affect every system in the body. It will also be vital to implement the stress-reducing techniques covered throughout this book as a way to restore your gut integrity and heal yourself from CFS. Are you beginning to see how *everything* in your body is linked? This is why nutritional and emotional health is so vital to recovery.

Fat is Your Friend

Given the fact your brain is more than 50% fat and that cholesterol is *required* in the methylation cycle which determines how every hormone, mineral and neurotransmitter functions within your body, your body *needs* fat in your diet. The myth that saturated fats are deadly was perpetuated in the 1980s with the pharmaceutical advent and promotion of "Statin" drugs, a myth that exists even today with many dieticians forced to conform to these out-dated guidelines if they wish to work in government sanctioned nutritionist roles in hospitals. The truth is, it is the *type* and *quality* of fat that is important, not the amount. Saturated fats from organic coconut oil, eggs, nuts, grass-fed meats, salmon and avocados are essential for many of your biological processes.

My food processor became my best friend in the kitchen when I had CFS, as I didn't have to spend any energy standing (which was difficult), chopping and mixing. Such activities would leave me unable to lift my arms for days. So I would simply tip dates, nuts, seeds, coconut oil, hemp protein, maple syrup and cacao into the food processor and press a button. Within a minute I had an organic nutritional powerhouse of protein, healthy fats, carbohydrates, minerals and vitamins I could simply roll into balls and take from the fridge as needed.

Good Bugs

By introducing fermented foods, healthy gut flora is encouraged to permeate your gut and settle your overworked immune system. Probiotics boost the mucosal immune system that protects the gastrointestinal tract and respiratory system and act as a shield to the outside world. This system is further protected by the systemic immune system, and studies are now showing that, by maintaining a healthy microbial gut balance with fermented foods and probiotics, the systemic immune response is boosted and inflammation markers are significantly reduced. If this balance is not maintained but is destroyed by stress, environmental toxins and poor diet, enzymes become altered, and your intestinal walls become permeable to toxins leeching into your system. This is a huge factor in CFS, with many sufferers showing signs of leaky gut syndrome and candida overgrowth. Correcting gut health with the addition of probiotics is necessary to strengthen your ability to protect yourself from microbes that can further weaken your already struggling system.

I began forcing sauerkraut into myself, initially gagging with every mouthful but telling myself it was all for the greater good! After a while I began to enjoy the salty morning routine, knowing I was supporting yet another aspect of my health in my journey to recovery. Start slowly when introducing fermented foods to your diet, as filling your gut with these good bugs can sometimes cause a die-off of the toxins that will leave you feeling a little worse. Over time though, you will wonder how you ever lived without these little magic helpers; your energy will increase, your mind will begin to clear and your moods will improve.

The importance of maintaining optimally healthy gut flora is now starting to finally pique the interest of researchers in treating mental health conditions such as autism, anxiety and even dementia. These would have normally been treated with pharmaceutical medications, but medical science is now beginning to acknowledge the key role intestinal microflora plays in controlling brain chemistry and inflammation.

The facts are, if you're eating pesticide-laden fruits and vegetables and processed foods, you're upsetting your gut chemistry as well as missing optimal nutrients from these altered, stored and "old" foods. Even if you are maintaining a clean diet, the fact that modern soils are now mineral-depleted means supplementation for many is necessary to both restore the health of the gut (and brain) and provide the necessary nutrients your body needs to restore you to full health.

Supplements

Because CFS is so complex, every individual will need different supplements at different times, and it is definitely advisable to gain the assistance of a naturopathic or functional medicine doctor in this regard. Vitamin, mineral and herbal supplements are used restoratively and as energy boosters and pain relievers. It is important to remember, though, that supplementation is not the cure, merely a vital part of the puzzle. Also, please be aware not everyone needs all of these supplements, and some interact with other medications in varying individuals, so only supplement under guidance. I buy most of my supplements through iherb.com as I can source high quality products far cheaper than retail and have them at my doorstep from the US to Australia within a week.

Listed in this chapter, in no particular order of importance, are the supplements I personally found most beneficial at various stages during my CFS journey to recovery.

B Group Vitmains:

Thiamine (B1)

Thiamine plays a key role in breaking down carbohydrates to produce energy, and as with all B vitamins, helps to maintain the nervous system. High dose supplementation usually isn't as necessary in CFS compared to some of the other B group vitamins, though it should be noted some foods and alcohol containing sulphites can inactivate any thiamine you are taking.

Riboflavin (B2)

This is the one that makes your pee bright yellow! A key vitamin in producing energy for the body, riboflavin also assists in the production of red blood cells, as well as activating B6 and folate in the body. B2 is essential for optimal functioning of the mitochondria and adrenals. It is also beneficial for migraines.

Niacin (B3)

Niacin is an essential vitamin for hormone production and the releasing of energy from fats, carbohydrates and proteins. For CFS sufferers, higher doses are best taken in the form of niacinamide, a pre-cursor to niacin that helps with building strength and decreasing fatigue. I temporarily took 500mg daily as recommended by Dr Sarah Myhill's protocol for supplementation to help restore mitochondrial function, though it is suggested to be wary of these doses if you have any liver issues.

Pantothenic Acid (B5)

Converted in the body to pantethine, B5 helps the body to better cope with stress because of the important role it plays in boosting healthy adrenal function. It helps the adrenals to become less sensitised to negative stress response. Had I known that I was progressing from adrenal fatigue to total adrenal exhaustion because of the stress my body was under in the years before the onset of CFS, I would have been taking at least 300mg daily of B5 and relaxing a lot more!

Pyridoxine (B6)

Pyridoxine is essential for a healthy nervous system and adrenal gland functioning. It contributes to making hormones and proteins, and is vital for manufacturing healthy neurotransmitter

Supplements

substances that carry signals in the brain. I take B6 in the activated pyridoxal 5-phosphate (P5P) form in a formula with zinc citrate, as I have a condition known as Pyroluria. This is a chemical imbalance involving an abnormality in hemoglobin synthesis that produces too much of a byproduct called kryptopyrrole. This byproduct binds to B6 and zinc in my body, removing them from my bloodstream, making these nutrients unavailable to perform the important physiological and chemical functions they would normally be used for.

Cobalamin (B12)

Essential for the production and regeneration of red blood cells as well as the growth of all cells, maintenance of a healthy gastrointestinal tract and nerves, B12, to me, has become the master vitamin. Without it in the methylcobalamin form at high doses, I don't think I would have begun to restore my health and energy to the level of functioning I have again now. This is due to my body being so depleted of it for a long time. B12 works with folate to help nerve cells to function optimally and also reduce levels of the inflammatory homocysteine in the blood.

Zinc

An essential trace element for immune system function, zinc also has a couple of rarely reported benefits specific to CFS, namely decreasing gut permeability and reducing tinnitus. It promotes anti-viral activity and is also a necessary mineral for adrenal function. Some forms of zinc can cause stomach upset and aren't easily absorbable, so it is advisable to obtain this supplement in picolinate or citrate form.

Coenzyme Q10

CoQ10 is an essential co-factor for energy production in the mitochondria along with D-Ribose and Carnitine, and is often severely depleted in CFS sufferers. CoQ10 helps reduce fatigue by stabilising muscle cell membranes and reducing muscle metabolism by-products that increase fatigue. It also boosts cardiac health. It is better utilised in ubidecarenone or ubiquinone forms rather that ubiquinol.

Vitamin D3

Vitamin D maintains healthy calcium balance in the body and is also very effective for mood regulation. The sun's rays trigger vitamin D synthesis, and nutritionally the best source is fresh coldwater fish. For CFS sufferers living in parts of the world experiencing short daylight hours in winter, supplementation may be necessary.

Vitamin A

Vitamin A, a fat-soluble vitamin, is essential for healing and proper immune function. It increases the body's resistance to infection, and helps the body to produce cells, effectively making it a necessary vitamin for overall well-being.

Vitamin E

Vitamin E is also a fat-soluble vitamin important in aiding the body's constant fight against oxidative stress. It reduces the free radical damage sustained by exercise and muscle exertion and boosts the immune system. It promotes healthy blood circulation and is helpful for the production and maintenance of red blood cells. It works in conjunction with glutathione to destroy free radicals.

Supplements

Vitamin C

Vitamin C is a potent detoxifier, antiviral, antioxidant, anti-allergen and strengthens the immune system. The body can tolerate very high levels of vitamin C, and some practitioners are even using IV vitamin C therapy as a "cure" for CFS, though with limited results. As you will come to learn, there are many elements you have to harmonise in your body and life in order to truly heal.

I found it extremely helpful to do Vitamin C "flushes" once a week. I still take 2000mg of ascorbic acid first thing of a morning to wake up my gut and get digestive enzymes flowing. However, in order to help rid your body of the toxic load it has accumulated over the years, and to counteract the current sluggish nature of your body's natural detoxification and methylation pathways as a CFS sufferer, doing a vitamin C flush with high levels of the vitamin can be helpful. Simply put, you take around 2000mg of vitamin C powder in water every 15 minutes for an hour or so until you reach what's called "tissue saturation"; that is, until you have watery diarrhoea. It wasn't fun, but it helped!

Probiotics

Because gut health is so critical when healing the body from CFS, a high quality probiotic is an essential supplement to counteract over-proliferation of unhealthy parasites, yeast and harmful microbes and the subsequent intestinal permeability. These friendly bacteria aid the body in digesting minerals and vitamins. A high quality probiotic supplement is a necessity when going through CFS, as levels of good bacteria are often low due to associated conditions such as leaky gut and candida. Most probiotic products will list the strains as well as numbers of living bacteria contained. Always choose one with live organism amounts of at least 10 billion. Fermented foods such as sauerkraut and kefir provide good bacteria to the gut as well.

Selenium

Selenium is a co-factor for the production of glutathione, and also a co-factor for thyroid hormone production. Its helps protect from free radical damage, and is immune boosting and anti-viral. Intake is dependent on selenium rich soils; otherwise, supplementation is necessary. Eating three or four organic Brazil nuts daily will also provide you with a boost of selenium.

Quercetin

Quercetin is a powerful bioflavinoid helping to stabilise cell membranes and also acts as an anti-histamine. It has anti-inflammatory properties and has been shown to reduce inflammatory cytokines. It is also beneficial for boosting mitochondria numbers in brain and muscle cells, protecting them from damage caused by the neurological deterioration, fatigue and cognitive problems CFS sufferers face.

Siberian Ginseng

Siberian Ginseng is an adaptogenic herb used to combat stress and fatigue. It provides a boost to the adrenal glands as well as the immune system, and I found it to be one of the more noticeably effective herbs for improving my energy levels and reducing the stress response. It can also help balance blood glucose levels and improve stamina and cognitive function.

Ashwaghanda (Withania)

Also known as Indian Ginseng, Withania is therapeutically used for nervous exhaustion, insomnia and adrenal stress. It is also

Supplements

an adoptogen, aiding the body's physiological systems in withstanding and reducing the immunosuppressive effects of stress. It is also used to treat anxiety, inflammatory conditions and neurological disorders.

Alpha Lipoic Acid

ALA is a sulphur-containing fatty acid and powerful anti-oxidant. It transforms glucose into energy in the mitochondria, and also helps protect the brain and central nervous system from free radical damage by mopping up oxidative stress. It also helps to recycle other antioxidants such as vitamin C, E and glutathione when they become depleted.

Ginko Biloba

Ginko Biloba leaf extract is a potent neuro-nutrient enhancing circulation, and is perfect for CFS sufferers to stimulate blood flow and detoxification pathways in the brain. It protects the brain from oxidative damage, increases cognitive and memory function and also helps to suppress the stress hormone, cortisol.

Slippery Elm

Used for healing inflamed tissues, this powdered bark protects and strengthens the digestive system, rapidly healing the gut wall, a vital component in healing from chronic illness. It has proven benefits for kidney, bladder and bowel inflammation.

Turmeric

Turmeric has so many health benefits it is now widely being touted as some newly discovered miracle spice! However, it has been used in Ayurvedic medicine for thousands of years to treat numerous ailments and aid longevity. In the case of CFS sufferers, turmeric is beneficial mostly for stimulating the production of what has been called "the master antioxidant", Glutathione. Because glutathione isn't effectively absorbed in supplement form and is often destroyed by stomach acids, it is necessary to stimulate the body's natural production mechanisms of glutathione.

Magnesium

Because not everyone will be eating five cups of organic leafy greens every single day, Magnesium is one of the body's most vital and often most depleted minerals. It is an essential nerve conductor and determines muscle function as well as over three hundred chemical reactions in the body. Your mitochondria need magnesium for optimal functioning. Muscle weakness, spasms, migraines and inflammation can all be addressed through magnesium supplementation.

I take various forms of the most absorbable magnesium, including magnesium malate, because it contains malic acid, which helps to clear lactic acid and stop muscle aches, magnesium citrate, and also spray on transdermal organic magnesium oil.

Chlorella and Chlorophyll

Both green plant substances that detoxify the body and supply it with an abundance of amino acids, proteins, enzymes and trace minerals, Chlorella and Chlorophyll make up part of my morning drink routine. Chlorella in particular binds to heavy metals in the digestive tract and removes them from the body. This is extremely useful for many people with CFS, where mercury toxicity can often be a contributing factor.

Essential Fatty Acids

Though I was initially recommended Evening Primrose Oil as a method of pain relief, I found little effect from it in that regard.

Supplements

There are numerous benefits, though, in taking a high quality evening primrose as well as fish oil supplement. Fish and flaxseed oils contain high levels of DHA and EPA and long-term use can offset the horrible migraines and joint and muscle pain experienced by so many CFS sufferers. EFA's are anti-inflammatory and immune boosting and high doses have also been shown to alleviate depression.

N-acetyl Carnitine

Carnitine levels in most CFS sufferers are extremely low and many holistic practitioners will recommend taking it as part of your supplement regime to treat CFS. It is essential for the conversion of fats into energy as well as delivering fatty acids into the mitochondria. I take the "n" form rather than the "l" form that is commonly recommended as N-acetyl Carnitine crosses the blood-brain barrier more effectively than L-acetyl Carnitine. I experienced increased cognition taking this supplement and still take it daily. It works with CoQ10 to enhance energy production.

L-Glutamine

Normally used by body builders to assist with the synthesis and protection of muscle tissue and the production of glycogen, glutamine is actually the most abundant amino acid in the body. Glutamine is something I used within my gut-healing regimen from the outset. It is fuel for healing enterocytes—the intestinal cells in the digestive tract—and can rapidly rectify leaky gut and inflammatory issues by nutritionally supporting the integrity of the intestinal lining.

N-acetyl Glucosamine (NAG)

NAG is an aminosaccharide, synthesised from glucose and

L-glutamine. It is excellent for joint health, but its health benefits for CFS sufferers can be attributed to its ability to heal the gut lining and promote the proliferation of healthy intestinal flora. It does this by forming a protective layer lining the digestive tract, and therefore enhances intestinal function. It is derived from shellfish, so caution is advised for those with seafood allergies.

Glutathione

Glutathione is known as the body's master antioxidant and primary detoxifying agent, and research shows that CFS sufferers are commonly deficient in this important protein molecule. It is also antiviral and antimicrobial, so raising glutathione levels in the body is essential for healing a system currently unable to effectively get rid of toxins. Supplementation orally is difficult, as the digestive system practically destroys it before cells can absorb it. Glutathione in the body can be boosted by taking its precursors N-acetyl Cysteine and Alpha Lipoic Acid, as well as undenatured whey protein and turmeric. Glutathione also works in conjunction with Vitamin E to destroy free radicals.

N-acetyl Cysteine (NAC)

An altered form of the amino acid Cysteine, NAC boosts the levels of the master antioxidant glutathione in the body, and has also been shown to strengthen the immune system by stimulating T-cells.

DHEA

DHEA (dehydroepiandrosterone) has been referred to as the "Mother Hormone", as it is a precursor to most other hormones. Replacing it when levels are shown to be low results in improved immune function, better stamina, regulated sleep and clearer cognition. It is widely used to overcome fatigue and immune issues and in the US is available over the counter as a sports supplement. Once I discovered the state my adrenals were in, I requested a tailored low dose DHEA and bioidentical cortisol supplement to begin to regulate my depleted hormonal system. It is important to note here that treating one aspect of CFS (in my case the adrenal and hormonal dysfunction) isn't just about supplementation, but the integration of individually ascertained and required levels of supplementation into your holistic recovery path. Not everyone with CFS will benefit from DHEA, as not everyone needs it. I did, and noticed improved sleeping patterns and improved cognition once my hormone levels began to stabilise and I applied the many other techniques throughout this book.

Astragalus

Astragalus is a powerful immune booster, commonly used in traditional Chinese medicine to support and stimulate energy flow. It aids heart function, and is a strong antiviral as well as a mild antibiotic. Astragalus strengthens the lungs where they are chronically weak.

D-Ribose

To make energy within the cells, your body needs to use a particular set of chemicals whose production is dependent on the presence of D-Ribose. D-Ribose is a complex sugar and is the catalyst that starts the metabolic process for the production of ATP (adenosine triphosphate), which is a co-enzyme carrying energy within the body's cells. Without D-Ribose, cells are unable to produce ATP, resulting in fatigue and lower energy levels. The introduction of D-Ribose into my supplement regime lifted my energy levels another notch from day one of starting it. I experienced improvements in my sleep, as well as a reduction in overall muscle pain.

Cat's Claw

Cat's Claw is a South American rainforest herb and is a potent anti-viral, anti-fungal, anti-bacterial and anti-inflammatory. It is useful for autoimmune conditions, allergies and for treating chronic and acute infections. It is used widely as part of the herbal Lyme healing protocol, though I took it for the aforementioned benefits.

Healthy Sleep

Healthy sleep is controlled by your natural body clock or circadian rhythm and the release of the hormone melatonin each night. Normally with circadian rhythm we are in a harmonic rhythm of activity and rest. Regular tiredness comes on at a certain time every night, as our natural rhythm starts to wind down and let our body know it's getting ready to sleep. Naturally we listen to our body and go to bed every night. Our nervous system regenerates and we wake up refreshed for the next day.

However, for we CFS sufferers it's an entirely different story! The circadian rhythm is a heavy metal drummer playing a 24-hour show at 300 beats per minute! There is no rotation of rest and activity, as the body does not cycle normally. This constant stress keeps our hypothalamus in overdrive, we miss our deep REM time, our hormones are constantly pumping out chemicals even as we "sleep", and consequently, we feel like we haven't slept for a month. Our methylation and detoxification systems begin to crash, our mitochondrial function dwindles and oxidative stress causes free radical damage because we have zero rejuvenation. We wake up like death rolled over to face another groundhog day of unrelenting fatigue.

This partly explains the "tired but wired" feeling that is common amongst CFS sufferers. In healthy bodies, the day is started with a higher level of cortisol that enables progression through the day. In CFS and cases of adrenal dysfunction, the morning cortisol level is almost negligible, which is why you start your day feeling like you have nothing in you. Because of your malfunctioning system, this cortisol slowly builds throughout the day to the point where it finally reaches a normal morning level or higher at night. This is why you can't sleep, much as you begin to feel like you're going to die if you don't get a proper night's rest. This cycle continues until addressed, managed and ultimately corrected.

Addressing the stress response is necessary to begin to break this pattern of insomnia and non-restorative sleep. I cover this information in another chapter if you wish to turn to this now. This is only one step to take to begin to sleep properly again and restore this balance. A number of factors helped me heal something that felt like it could have driven me crazy at one point, something that is so crucial to every aspect of recovery and a necessity for living a long and healthy life in general. Sleep and rest time must become a healing state.

Turn off Screens at Night Time

As a CFS sufferer I found my iPhone was at times my only (lonely) connection to a world I was no longer a part of. When lying there I was often reading some research articles, watching YouTube videos or messaging with friends in very short bursts. However, the constant and repeated night time zombie phone pattern actually stops the body producing melatonin, the chemical needed that tells your body it's time for sleep, and increases the production of cortisol. For someone afflicted with CFS whose cortisol levels are beginning to rise at night anyway because of your malfunctioning adrenal glands (that tired but wired feeling), the last thing you want to be doing is further exacerbating the problem just from staring at a screen. Blue-lit screens such

Healthy Sleep

as those in phones, laptops and tablets completely disrupt your circadian rhythm. There are apps you can buy which change the colour of your screen light as well as physical filters to attach to your screens. However, the easiest solution is simply to not use any screens for a few hours before you wish to sleep and instead, begin to apply some of the other helpful pre-sleeping rituals discussed here.

To restore your circadian rhythm, the most effective solution is to get morning light. As soon as you can in the morning, get in the sun, and if that's not possible, open a window to allow natural light in. This sends an immediate signal to your body clock to reset and wake up. As I experienced photosensitivity a lot during CFS, this was a challenge for me. But you only need a few minutes to begin with, and as you become more desensitised to light and your body begins to regulate as you sleep better, you can increase your morning light exposure time. This technique also regulates your metabolism, digestion, hormonal levels and body temperature, helping you to lose weight and more effectively absorb nutrients from food and supplements.

Do Restorative Yoga Before Sleep

Restorative yoga poses can be extremely helpful in promoting a restful sleep. When I was pretty much bed-bound, the term "yoga pose" struck fear into my heart. I could barely move, and someone suggested I do restorative yoga poses for ten minutes before sleep. However, these poses are very simple, non-straining and aided by pillows. The meditative aspect of yoga combined with deep breathing and gentle restorative postures work to calm your stress response. The parasympathetic nervous system is activated during restorative yoga, which moves your body and mind out of the sympathetic nervous system response it has become stuck in.

Your adrenals will become relaxed and return to optimal functioning again. Over time your biochemistry is altered (in a good way!) providing you with therapeutic sleep, rather than wired, stressful and broken nights where your brain won't even let you enter the healing alpha state of sleep.

There are three restorative yoga poses I found helpful for inducing a more restful sleep and calming my racing mind:

Legs up the Wall: lie in front of a wall or chair, lifting your legs straight up the wall or resting on the chair. Place a pillow under your head and allow your arms to open out to the side. Breathe.

Seated Forward Bend: Sit with legs extended or crossed and place pillows on your legs. Allow your head to rest forward comfortably on the pillow, your arms relaxed by your side. Breathe.

Child's Pose: Sit on your heels with a pillow placed in front of you. You can also place a pillow between your hips and heels. Rest your head forward onto the pillow; turn your head to one side and arms by your side relaxed backward. Like a baby having a rest. Breathe.

Be sure to continually return your focus to your breathing as you allow thoughts to come and go. It is also vital you practice diaphragmatic, or "belly" breathing. This is something to practice and maintain throughout your daily life as well, because the bad habit of shallow chest breathing continually drip feeds stress hormones into your system. These poses can be held for 10-15 minutes each. Even if you can only rest in one pose for 10 minutes each night, over time you will begin to notice positive changes to your ability to enter deeper sleep.

Healthy Sleep

4/7/8 Breathing Technique

Now that I have recovered from CFS, I tend to sleep like a baby! I get to bed about 10 pm feeling naturally tired, and within 10 minutes I'm sound asleep. I wake up around 6 am and get into the sun. However, I still have the odd night where I wake up at 3 am needing to pee, or have some negative emotions still swimming around from my day, causing me to lay in bed awake and think. This breathing technique is the one thing that still works for me, hands down, every single time I feel I can't switch off and get to sleep and was something I began to practice during my CFS insomnia.

It is simply breathing in for a 4-count, holding the breath for a 7-count and breathing out slowly and gently for an 8-count. The technique elicits calm and relaxation, filling the circulatory system with oxygen and acts as a natural sedative for the nervous system. Literature suggests one can fall asleep in under a minute using this technique, and indeed I have, though it does take some practice to relax into the rhythm of the technique and not focus on the counting.

Testing: The Hidden Factors

The immune system that is improperly activated uses an immense amount of energy. Given the amount of energy your body uses just to function, an excessive load on the immune system wastes energy that you simply don't have to waste. In the example of an allergy (wheat, dairy or mould) your immune system is on overdrive, taking up a large chunk of your body's energy. The immunity of your body becomes depressed from overwork, leading to persistent infections, allergic reactions and food and chemical intolerances. Thus, it is wise to begin to search for hidden sites of chronic infection, possible hormonal imbalances, recurring viruses and areas of gut infection and dysfunction to switch this overdrive off.

It's a ridiculous statement to have to make but it's true—finding a general practitioner openly willing to order relevant tests in the early stages of you presenting with any manner of seemingly unexplainable ongoing illness will be a challenge. An overwhelming majority of doctors no longer look for causes, nor do they take the time and effort to accurately diagnose, as there simply isn't time to do so! For a medical system in collective denial of invisible illnesses, don't be surprised if your concerns are met with condescension and apathy. It took me countless doctor's appointments and over nine months of suffering before I discovered myself I should have had an adrenal test and then went and demanded one. Lo and behold, my adrenals were functioning

Testing: The Hidden Factors

at about 10% of a healthy person and my morning cortisol level was almost nil!

As tempting as it is to raise the middle finger at this system, you need a medical doctor (and preferably a naturopathic doctor and functional medicine physician) to order and assess all of these tests. This is only the beginning of the healing journey to both rule out other possible causes of symptoms, as well as to find markers that may have led to CFS. You will also find it beneficial to seek help from a chiropractor, nutritionist, acupuncturist and counsellor. You must become pro-active, take matters into your own hands and direct your healing path.

This may seem disheartening and complex, especially when you are bedridden, but taking control of your path to recovery requires educating yourself on all possible avenues and then walking down each one. These are the basic starting points in finding answers and treatment options. Some of these tests are free, some will have costs that vary from country to country, but all are essential to knowing exactly how your body is functioning at this point in time. Some CFS sufferers spend years in horrible fatigue, as their basic Thyroid Stimulating Hormone levels indicate a normally functioning thyroid; they trusted this information and went home to bed, when, in fact, further investigation into a complete Thyroid Hormone Profile may have given a clearer indication of dysfunction explaining fatigue levels, finally indicating they needed supplementation and thus, relief from some symptoms as a pathway to healing was uncovered and acted upon.

It is common for the standard full blood count in CFS sufferers to be normal, hence the label you've been cursed with, as most doctors don't know what else to call it to summarise your symptoms! However, you must trust your instincts and insist on the following tests:

Adrenal Hormone Profile

CFS is so much more than a cortisol problem, but severe adrenal exhaustion is something I was clinically diagnosed with after more than nine months of flailing in the darkness of a hopeless medical system, so it was definitely a co-factor in contributing to the level of suffering I was experiencing. It should have been my doctors leading this discussion, not myself, after having already endured symptoms for so much time, just barely being able to walk to the toilet and back.

For the years leading up to my CFS crash, I was overworked, overstressed and overtraining. The most common signs of adrenal fatigue, such as trouble sleeping, continued exhaustion, salt and sugar cravings, decreased ability to handle stress, light-headedness, nervousness, poor memory, allergies, trouble getting out of bed and being prone to flu gradually became a regular part of my existence. Despite many doctor visits that often resulted in yet another antibiotic script for yet another "viral infection" that the antibiotic wouldn't actually treat, nobody once mentioned the stages of adrenal fatigue to me. By the time I had my first adrenal test nine months following a CFS diagnosis (the diagnosis of which can only "officially" be given after more than six months of living like this!), I was diagnosed as late stage adrenal exhaustion—the final stage where cortisol production drops to levels insufficient to maintain any kind of normal physiological function.

The adrenals determine the adjustment of energy delivery to demand. My demand well exceeded delivery, and I was in trouble!

Testing: The Hidden Factors

Your adrenal glands sit just above the kidneys and produce adrenaline, noradrenaline, aldosterone, dehydroepiandrosterone (DHEA) and cortisol. Adrenaline and cortisol are your body's first line of chemical defence when placed under stress. Too much stress, whether physical, emotional or environmental, causes overworking of your adrenals, as well as dysfunction in your hypothalamus-pituitary-adrenal (HPA) axis from the continual overproduction of cortisol. This unbalanced state leads to adrenal exhaustion, where cortisol production is negligible, resulting in the loss of many basic functions and increased inflammation. Your hypothalamus is constantly activated, your sympathetic nervous system engaged and you remain stuck in a flight-or-fight response.

Modern medicine only really recognises adrenal fatigue at its most extreme form as Addison's disease. The delays in diagnosis and treatment of adrenal fatigue thus cause unnecessary suffering, longer recovery time and the consequent "burden" on the system. Ironically, this is the very burden many doctors try to avoid by cost-saving measures of not actually ordering tests, instead of doing so and following up with suitable holistic treatments or lifestyle advice. Adrenal fatigue is easily and immediately diagnosable and treatable with supplements and stress reduction techniques. So why must people all around the world suffer from varying levels of medical incompetence?

So, to avoid unnecessary suffering, get numbers! Demand a full Adrenal Hormone Profile Test. It involves collecting saliva samples at four times throughout the day and sending them back to a lab. Simple! This measures your cortisol production and secretion throughout the day as well as oestrone (e1), oestradiol (e2), progesterone, dhea-s and testosterone. Everyone with adrenal exhaustion will have differing hormonal levels of dysfunction, and for that reason, each individual must be assessed for their unique hormonal needs for supplementation. Because my cortisol production was almost nil, I requested and was prescribed bioidentical hydrocortisone and DHEA until further tests showed I was beginning to restore my adrenal functioning.

As well as overwork and environmental toxins, emotional tiredness will always cause a drain on adrenal function. This cannot be addressed by physical rest, but rather by addressing the patterns in your response that *allows* this to happen. It is pointless correcting a biological imbalance in the form of a supplement without addressing the emotional root. Adrenal issues can often manifest because of unresolved or long-standing life issues. You must stop giving away your power to others and act according to your own inner truth. You must begin to become present and aware of when you lose your equanimity and begin to rush. Rushing and overthinking may feel normal, but it is not a normal state to be in. Yet in today's world, it's the state everyone seems to function in! You must remove stress from your life and learn to respond differently to any stress that does occur. Contained herein is a wealth of information based on my own learning and experience you can apply to help heal your stress response.

Complete Thyroid Profile

Hypothyroidism is something worth testing for in your quest for answers, as thyroid disorders can mimic many symptoms of CFS, such as breathlessness, fatigue, numb extremities, severe muscle cramps, frequent infections, cognitive issues and digestive problems. A slow thyroid will make you feel sluggish and lethargic, as

Testing: The Hidden Factors

the thyroid hormone thyroxine regulates many activities in your body.

Most doctors will only ever order the standard Thyroid Stimulating Hormone (TSH) test to check your thyroid, and this will probably come back within normal range, despite you presenting with all the symptoms of an underactive thyroid. This is because normal range is a population average taken from a narrow section of the healthy population, which is basically irrelevant to what your particular functional levels should and will be as a CFS sufferer.

Therefore, it is essential you order a complete thyroid profile to cover TSH, free T4, Free T3, Reverse T3, Thyroid Peroxidase Antibodies (TPOAb) and Thyroglobulin Antibodies (TgAb). These particular tests assess whether precursor hormones are being converted into their active forms, inactive transport forms, and if you have a dysfunctional gland making "reverse T3" which is essentially applying a brake pedal to your body.

The adrenal and thyroid glands work together in producing their corresponding hormones. Quite often, addressing an adrenal issue will correct a thyroid issue, without the need for thyroid hormone intervention, whilst conversely, ignoring an adrenal problem can have a negative cascading effect on the thyroid gland. Thus, it is necessary to test thyroid function in conjunction with adrenal function. If adrenal function has decreased, the thyroid responds by producing more thyroid hormones to compensate. By overcompensating for adrenal insufficiency, this overload of thyroid hormones can also attribute to the tired but wired symptoms. If left running at such a rate, the thyroid can burn out and hyperthyroidism can result. Also, if treating thyroid hormones without addressing adrenal issues, thyroid medications can actually aggravate adrenal stress.

Viral Infections

With the body stuck in overdrive and susceptible to infectious agents, the immune cells, which would ordinarily have a regular response, begin to excessively produce antibodies (which attack the infectious agent) and release alarm chemicals, called cytokines, and recruit other immune cells to fight. The trouble is, these alarm cells act on other cells as well, particularly those that affect your brain and muscles, and they can go further into alarm mode. They decrease energy usage, and therefore you become unusually fatigued. Because there's less "electricity", there's less production, so you get loss of basic function, can't remember things, you feel like your brain doesn't work properly and you can't walk very far. When the electricity in your body is turned off for too long, you can develop cell injury. Normally, the infection would burn out after about four weeks, yet the nature of CFS keeps you trapped in this state due to the vicious cycle of immune deregulation. Latent viral infections are seemingly constantly re-triggered and new viruses invade our compromised systems.

The most commonly tested-for viral infections found in CFS patients are:

Epstein-Barr virus (EBV) or human herpes virus 4 (HHV4),
Cytomegalovirus (CMV) or human herpes virus 5 (HHV5),
Human herpes virus 6 (HHV6),
Herpes simplex virus 1 and 2 (HSV1 and HSV2),
Varicella-zoster virus or chickenpox, and
Coxsackie virus

Testing: The Hidden Factors

Whilst blood tests will indicate whether you have antibodies from a previous viral infection (meaning you've had a particular virus before) or are currently fighting one, there is little you can do to isolate and repair this one aspect of your body alone, as a whole body approach to healing is required. By regaining homeostasis through a whole body healing approach to recovery, recurring viruses will no longer be an issue.

Lyme Disease

Lyme Disease is a tick-borne infection presenting many symptoms that mimic CFS. Lyme in the initial and immediate stages is treated effectively with a few weeks of antibiotics. When it is left undiagnosed, or misdiagnosed as CFS, it leaves sufferers to go for years with the bacteria eating away at their cells, becoming Chronic Lyme. Some people endure many years of antibiotic treatment to little avail, and some have had great success using the Buhner Protocol, a system of herbal anti-bacterials to destroy the Lyme bugs and co-infections. People are also having success using bee venom through Apitherapy to kill the Borrelia bacteria and cysts.

Lyme isn't something I was afflicted with, and therefore isn't an area I personally know a lot about, though I did do some research into it as I was told it might be a possible reason for all of my CFS symptoms. However, there is no testing available in Australia for Lyme and at $2k to send bloods to the US to risk getting back a false result (which is apparently common), it wasn't something I could afford to do.

But Lyme doesn't exist in Australia. Nor does it exist in the US, the UK or anywhere. That is, according to your medical boards and governments! It is a joke and an atrocity their collective heads are either buried in the sand or firmly stuck somewhere else, to be dismissive of one of the world's most prevalent environmental bacterial infections which devastates so many lives. And no government would want to acknowledge the prevalence of an epidemic because that costs money and would be an admission of the mistreatment of so many people. If you aren't a politician and actually live in the real world and can obtain a test result clearing you of Lyme disease, I urge you to do so. The sooner treatment is started if you're infected, the better your outcome.

Gut Integrity

The path to thriving health always starts with the gut, as its function is to break down what we feed ourselves to nourish every cell in our body. The old adage "you are what you eat" isn't just a marketing catch phrase, but a quite literal description that what we consume becomes who we are physically. At one point in my life I'm surprised I didn't turn into a Snickers bar! With my health restored and my diet clean I can joke now, but mostly I just shake my head in dismay at my former self for what I did to my gut and consequently, my entire system, with poor diet, medications and stress.

I had regularly overused non-steroidal anti-inflammatory drugs (NSAIDs) to treat a back injury, uninformed of any implications of long-term use. By switching off the restorative proteins, NSAIDs actually block the gut's ability to naturally heal, ironically causing chronic inflammation of the intestinal lining, intestinal permeability and an inability to effectively absorb nutrients from food and supplements. After experiencing constant stomach pain and nausea for a while, I was diagnosed by gastroscopy with duodenitis, inflammation of the duodenum, and placed on the proton pump inhibitor Somac, which had further dire consequences for my digestive tract, compounding an already sensitive and damaged system!

It is not uncommon for the CFS sufferer to unknowingly have compromised gut integrity from dysbiosis caused by toxins, diet, oral contraceptives or frequent antibiotic use, which leads to candida, then leaky gut and a plethora of tumbling health issues that can contribute to many CFS symptoms. Starting a clean diet, removing allergenic foods, sugars and alcohol, reducing stress and environmental contaminants are just the beginning. To begin your healing journey, you must assess if any of the above issues which could be compromising your digestive health are relevant to you through the following tests:

Comprehensive Digestive Stool Analysis

As the name implies, this is the most comprehensive digestive health and function test to begin with. It will determine candida levels, harmful microbes as well as levels of good bacteria in the gut. Your digestive health is measured by your gut's ability to break down carbohydrates, proteins and fats and this test will provide an accurate assessment of how your digestive system is operating. If candida is found to be present, the best solution is to permanently remove the cause – usually sugars, grains, alcohol and pharmaceuticals. Anti-fungal and natural remedies like Olive Leaf Extract, Pau D'Arco, Oregano Oil, Garlic, Acidophilus and Bifidus bacteria and Cat's Claw can also be useful, but expect a temporary Herxheimer reaction as die-off of the bacteria occurs with any candida treatment.

Heliobacter Pylori Test

The single biggest cause of stomach ulcers and cancer apart from stress, these bacteria can remain hidden, giving you some nasty abdominal symptoms. If found, it is usually treated by doctors with a triple combination of antibiotics, antiparasitic drugs and protein pump inhibitors, all of which have their own harmful effects on other aspects of gut health. Medicinal grade Manuka

Gut Integrity

Honey has also been proven to kill H. pylori as well as heal stomach ulcers and intestinal inflammation.

Parasitology Screening

If you've ever travelled, had children in day-care or drunk from a water tank, chances are you've met a parasite! Giardia is most commonly found, and can present as not only digestive, but also neurological symptoms. As always, pharmaceuticals will be prescribed, further upsetting intestinal balance and weakening an already overburdened liver. Herbal remedies for parasitic infections include Garlic, Golden Seal and Grape Seed Extract. Chiropractic intervention is also extremely effective, as a good chiropractor will work from a whole body approach to healing, often starting with techniques testing gut health.

Intestinal Permeability Test

This test is the most effective for determining if you have leaky gut syndrome. Intestinal permeability occurs when the intestinal walls become so weakened that toxic chemicals leak through it and into the bloodstream, activating your immune response to fight the particles. You then become sensitised to foods and environmental substances. That is also a common CFS trait, your body living in a constant state of immune response, inflammation and heightened stress.

L-Glutamine and N-acetyl Glucosamine were the main supplements I took for healing and restoring my gut function, along with a daily morning dose of ascorbic acid and Bragg's organic apple cider vinegar to essentially "wake up" and increase my digestive acids to promote nutrient absorption. The herbs Slippery Elm and Aloe Vera are also highly effective in repairing the mucosal lining.

The MTHFR of a Mutation!

Generally speaking, I've been an anxious person my entire life, worrying about "what ifs", and throwing up before I went onstage to play a gig. Everyone has their funny quirks, and I just thought these must be mine! Little did I know, a rather common genetic mutation with a simple mineral supplement solution my body was lacking could have caused me a life of anxiety.

It is called methylenetetrahydrofolate reductase (MTHFR, suitably!) and, put simply, my body is unable to convert folic acid into a form I can use effectively. My MTHFR gene has inherited a homozygous or double mutation at the location of C677T, predisposing me to high levels of homocysteine. This simple flaw in my system went undetected until recently, and in many, it is an undiscovered cause of much of the anxiety that anxiety-prone people seem to live with. It has also definitely contributed to some of my health problems throughout my life, because of the breakdown of the methylation pathways so critical for detoxification and neurological functioning.

With regards to CFS, the MTHFR gene mutation will not cause CFS and supplementing will not cure it, but it is indeed another necessary link to uncover in the puzzle to whole body healing, because healthy methylation is critical in so many bodily functions – it turns genes on and off, repairs DNA, makes glutathione, detoxifies chemicals and heavy metals, builds immune cells, reduces histamine, processes hormones, repairs cell membranes, supports neurotransmitters, turns the stress response on

The MTHFR of a Mutation!

and off and helps our energy cycle create carnitine, CoQ10 and ATP to support mitochondrial energy.

A properly functioning MTHFR gene synthesizes folate into a specific form needed to turn the toxic metabolite homocysteine into methionine, which is essential for cell growth and DNA metabolism. Methionine is also used by your body to make proteins, utilize antioxidants and assist your liver to process fats. Methionine is converted in your liver into adenosylmethionine, also known as SAM-e, a natural metabolite of methionine in the body. Because SAM-e helps produce, then break down your brain chemicals serotonin, dopamine and melatonin, a deficiency of methionine leads to reduced levels of SAM-e and an increased risk of depression. To bypass this, I now need to take L-5-methyltetrahydrofolate (5-mthf), the bioavailable form of folic acid and methylcobalamin B12 to assist my body in methylating correctly.

However, I found that kickstarting my methylation process after a lifetime of my body compensating for this under functioning system was not without risk. My body was thrown into instant detoxification, and the initial neurological side effects were quite a shock. Consequently, the process often requires further genome testing to assess disruption in any other methylation pathways, and professionally guided trial and error to find a personalized supplement dose before the methylation pathways are again operating correctly. So be sure to investigate and treat this only under the guidance of a good chiropractic, naturopathic or functional medicine doctor. They are YOUR genes after all!

Chiropractic Care

The benefits of chiropractic care cannot be understated. On both a physical and emotional level, chiropractic sessions have enabled me to become educated about living a holistic life. I have literally been adjusted to live well and thrive.

Chiropractic focuses on the nervous system, and through various techniques a good chiropractor can interrupt, correct and re-energise a dysfunctional nervous system, freeing you from pain, fatigue, cognitive dysfunction and digestive issues. The stuck energy is unblocked and cleared, and the nervous system is able to function effectively again. Finding a good chiropractor is one of the most beneficial actions you can take, for not only your health and healing journey from CFS, but also the long-term health of your family. I have gained more healing and knowledge about my body from my chiropractors than any general practitioner, the only exception being a cherished functional medicine doctor whose assistance and advice has also been invaluable.

Chiropractic is probably the most under-rated and belittled whole body healing profession that exists today. It is a practice that, despite it's proven scientific benefits, is constantly under attack by the medical profession. Chiropractors are forced to publicly defend the effectiveness and relevance of their industry in the vortex of a mainstream media-controlled and corporatized health system where pharmaceutical companies dictate policy for the benefit of themselves and shareholders. In Australia, a lobby group of high profile doctors called the Friends of Science

Chiropractic Care

in Medicine (FSM) is campaigning to have "alternative medicine" degrees like chiropractic, naturopathy, homeopathy, Chinese medicine, kinesiology, reflexology and osteopathy removed from Australian universities under the guise these professions "put the public at risk." It is a tragedy that the integrity of these modalities is publicly maligned by self-serving groups like this, as well as organisations such as the Australian National Health and Medical Research Council (NHMRC), who also seek to discredit their scientific and holistic health benefits.

These unfortunate truths aside, two amazing chiropractors have helped my health and my life immeasurably over the years. Using their chiropractic techniques, combined with traditional body modification, kinesiology, cranial osteopathy, emotional healing and some really painful tendon loosening poking at times, I have felt energetic changes in me literally from the moment I've left the practice. I had presented at times almost being unable to walk; my head feeling like it were stuffed with cotton wool; being riddled with pain; feeling like my brain was three steps behind me and have left feeling like I could take on the world. I definitely credit a lot of my restored health from my back injury, gut issues and energy disorders to the healing powers of my chiropractors, and I am forever grateful for the effectiveness of the profession physically, emotionally and educationally.

Bounce!

Once you have progressed past the acute stage of CFS and can tolerate movement that is a bit more vigorous, I highly recommend buying a rebounder or mini-trampoline. Rebounding is one of the most effective forms of exercise, and has numerous benefits for CFS patients. The movement benefits the immune system by increasing lymphatic drainage and detoxifying the body. In CFS sufferers, the sympathetic nervous system becomes overloaded and begins to decrease blood flow and lymphatic drainage. This causes further toxins to accumulate, and a vicious cycle ensues, with long-term irritation of the sympathetic nervous system weakening an already frail immune system even further. Rebounding is one of the best ways to help drain toxins from the nervous system by stimulating healthy lymph flow.

The motion stimulates internal organs, boosting immunity and improving digestion. It also moves the cerebral spinal fluid, as well as the aqueous fluid in your eyes, naturally improving eyesight. The obvious side effects of reduced body fat and improved balance are great, but I think the most significant benefit to come from rebounding is the fact it has been shown to improve the mitochondria count within cells, thereby reducing fatigue and improving endurance. Complete inactivity can have physiological consequences, as the total number of mitochondria is dependant on levels of movement. If you can aim for a minute to start, and increase to five minutes a few times a week, you will begin to notice a change in your energy levels and strength as I did.

Cold Shower Therapy

Cold Shower Therapy

Sometimes I'm sure the neighbours really do wonder what all the shrieking is, coming from next door every morning. I have a cold shower every single day. Whilst I live in the beautiful sunny Gold Coast in Queensland, Australia, it's not always warm weather and not always how I want to start my day. But I do it anyway.

I began having cold showers during some of the worst of my CFS symptoms because I had read about some of the health benefits, like improved immunity and enhanced muscle recovery. I was willing to try anything. Having cold showers helps increase circulation and lymphatic drainage, and I definitely noticed and still continue to notice an improvement physically from having them. I feel better immediately after having one, no matter how I was feeling when I got in.

I think what appeals to me most about cold shower therapy, though, is the psychological aspect. Picture this: it's a chilly winter morning and you stumble into the bathroom. The last thing you want to do is have a cold shower. The mere thought of the freezing needles of water blasting your skin is petrifying. You turn the cold tap and hesitate. Then comes that snap decision, that second of bravery where you tell yourself "I can do this." And in you go! It fucking sucks! Your body almost convulses in shock. Sounds come from your mouth like a primal animal as you turn and shiver and punch away imaginary attackers. After about a minute of this primitive freak-out, something happens.

AWAKEN WELLNESS

You become immune to everything that was happening just before and start to focus on your breath. It becomes almost meditational, standing there under the freezing water. You are here now in your stillness and it is blissful. You turn off the tap and dry off. You did what felt unassailable, and because you did, you know you can do it again tomorrow. The funny part is, tomorrow morning you will be met with the same inner resistance, the same hesitation and fear. With that instant of resolve, you'll dive in again. Every day you will grow stronger as you push through another barrier. Soon you begin to know deep within that you can face and do anything.

Developing emotional resilience is one factor that is crucial for healing the broken body, and cold showers actually train your body to become more resilient to stress. Also, doing something you are mentally resistant to on a daily basis takes a lot of will power. Over time you become disciplined in maintaining this habit and your ability to plunge headlong into anything you face becomes a more automatic response throughout all areas of your life. Anything you can do to contribute to reducing and reframing your stress response will eventually lead you on the path to healing your body and brain from CFS.

The Broken Brain

The Broken Brain

For many months before my CFS diagnosis, I was in a state of debilitating cognitive decline. This would last in its most severe unrelenting form for at least another year. I had enrolled to study Nursing at university, and was doing creative copywriting and pursuing entrepreneurial ventures. I found study and knowledge acquisition easy and took for granted my intelligence and ability to jump into any field and apply myself to it. I have wide and varying interests, so I have studied a lot and lived many "careers" in my lifetime, sometimes several at once. I could research and write an essay in a day; if I heard a song once I could play it, and I was fond of dabbling in trying to learn numerous languages.

Consequently, when CFS hit me, I couldn't fathom my instant cognitive regression. I could no longer read, and when I could it was in five-minute blocks, sometimes only one per day. I could no longer write some days, and when I did had forgotten how to spell. This was incomprehensible for a former copywriter! My mouth wouldn't form the words my brain wanted to say, and I would often speak how a person with dyslexia writes, with jumbled sentence structure. It upset me so much that some days I couldn't listen to my girls' voices, nor could I interpret what they were saying. My brain became so slow at processing information and combined with no memory whatsoever, there were times I thought I might have early onset dementia! I would leave the stove on and put the TV remote in the fridge! I had no concept of time and some days had to think hard to remember the names I had given my children when I wanted to call out to them. That was soul crushing.

My stress response was so heightened I could physically feel stressful energy like a weight smothering me. I became overwhelmed with a blockage of trapped emotional energy holding onto incidences where friends and family had screwed me over. I internalised it all and held onto the anger and frustration, both with them and with myself, believing there was some great fault in me that caused people to attack me in such a way. My system was in such a hyper-alert state, I lived with visual disturbances, flashing colours and extreme light and sound sensitivity. I required darkness and silence just to survive. "Differential activation" is the term for when your body becomes hyper reactive to everything – light, medications, sound, foods, triggers – your body is so hyper aroused it wants to get away from any triggers, as it simply can't deal with life. This is something I found was one of the most terrifying aspects of CFS.

With time and practice (and it takes a lot of both), I learnt this is something you can turn off by conditioning a new emotional response to stress and triggers. Understanding the physiology of emotional stress it absolutely vital in healing from CFS.

The Physiology of Emotional Stress

It is commonly noted among CFS sufferers that a pattern of chronic physical, emotional or environmental stress together with a physiological trigger causes the descent. A hyper alert response strikes in the hypothalamus, which becomes locked in defence mode. In my case, it was exactly that perfect recipe of the aforementioned constant stress combination and the final viral result. The body is primarily concerned with survival. It doesn't care how you feel physically; it's just trying to keep you alive! So this response is constantly reacting in the background with your limbic system thinking it has to continually defend against a threat.

The hypothalamus is the master gland in the body, responsible for producing hormones that stimulate the release and regulation of other hormones in the body. Corticotropin-releasing hormone (CRH) stimulates adrenocorticotropic-releasing hormone (ACTH) by the pituitary gland, which in turn stimulates the adrenals to produce cortisol. If the hypothalamus goes into a state of overdrive from being in a perpetual environment of psychological or physiological stress, the body's entire endocrine system malfunctions, eventually leading to many of the symptoms experienced by CFS sufferers.

Perpetuation of this vicious cycle occurs as your Sympathetic Nervous System (SNS) is constantly aroused, causing adrenal exhaustion, oxidative stress, latent virus reactivation, more allergies and chemical sensitivities and mitochondrial dysfunction.

The Broken Brain

The constant triggering of your SNS is battling your immune system, and they work in a vicious cycle, perpetuating the hell you struggle to exist in called CFS!

As the brain is hyper sensitised, the information it is taking in because of all of these horrible symptoms causes it to think it is still in danger, and therefore it restimulates the SNS, triggering more symptoms and furthering the condition. The hippocampus shrinks from this process and is unable to switch off the sympathetic response. Pioneering UK CFS researcher Dr Sarah Myhill likens it to an out of control car with no brakes! The entire brain is now completely stuck in this hyper arousal state and unable to switch off. This is why you feel so completely debilitated and empty, unable to perform even the most basic functions in your daily life.

When you're stuck in this state, you lose sight of all the things you can do that could help you. When your life has been (to put it mildly) completely disordered by CFS, it is very easy to become consumed with sick person thoughts. Your life is so restricted and limited now compared to the one you were living prior to becoming so ill, and so every thought, action and future event becomes one of survival. Because we are stuck in a state of perceiving threats (in this case the threat feels like our own body turning against us) we are continually and unknowingly training our hypothalamus to be constantly fearful. It becomes sensitised to everything, almost to the point where the response is irrational.

Therefore we constantly worry about "being ill". This shitty illness has put our lives on hold—even taken away our lives in many cases. Symptoms are seen as a curse, and this perpetual negativity about our bodies, the irritation of never getting better and the constant frustration with not being able to do what we really want continues to reinforce in your hypothalamus that something is wrong! This constant perception of danger or that something is wrong means more and more stress hormones are released, further straining the sympathetic nervous system and thus, more symptoms occur. This creates a vicious cycle where all of this mental stress results in the body feeling like it has physically run a marathon. The body reacts to its own reactions and becomes so highly sensitive that any situation where you may be expected to expend energy in any way becomes an impossibly fearful one.

I know all too well the feeling of helplessness that comes when you face another heavy day. However, there are so many tools that, once understood and combined, will allow you to write your own prescription for healing. If you can heal this response and begin to own your emotional reaction to this cavalcade of symptoms, this becomes a powerful differentiator between whether you set yourself on the path to healing and whether your body and brain remains stuck in this state.

Healing the Broken Brain

What's amazing about this broken system is the fact that this debilitating physiological conditioning is determined by and can eventually be healed by emotional response. Your response to your symptoms can either heal or perpetuate this illness. Brains are neuroplastic and completely able to be rewired. This condition is not in the mind, *but it is in the brain*. I can remember feeling so disgusted and insulted by a doctor who told me CFS was all in my mind and to just eat vegetables and get out more. I was mocked, and being unable to effectively communicate in my dyslexic cognitive state, I was emotionally defeated by a seemingly superior intellect. This negative experience alone caused me to crash heavily, as I spiralled further into a state of heightened stress, feeling like the professionals being paid to help find answers for what I was going through weren't willing or able to do anything at all. I stressed about the symptoms of yet another horrible crash and more weeks spent in bed and thus, the cycle continued. I knew there had to be another way and this had to stop. I already ate vegetables every day!

When there is a threat, there is a physiological response, an immune response and an emotional response. All are intertwined. By emotionally reducing the perception of threat, you are able to reduce the response by the brain to any stress. You must retrain yourself to respond to life completely differently from how you have been up until this point. Every time you train and reinforce a new response, you are rewiring your brain, healing your stress response and the entire hormonal cascade throughout your body adjusts to your new way of being. It takes more than just affirmations and positive thinking alone; it takes action, visualisation and actually *feeling* how you want to feel. It takes discipline and repeated sustained effort to achieve this gradual alleviation of the condition. It is a whole body state change. The human condition as a whole must be looked at in order to heal. Chronic illness can originate from any level of mind, body and spirit, and you must examine the possible causes of symptoms from every one of these levels in order to understand what they are telling you. And then you must listen and take action!

By mastering your thoughts and only filling your mind with empowering statements and beliefs, you will begin to make choices more in line with what you want. These choices will lead to wider experiences giving you positive emotional rewards. In the case of a CFS sufferer, your thoughts may be about wanting to be better. Not only do you want to feel better, you want to feel vibrant, brimming with energy and overflowing with vitality and joyous enthusiasm for every moment you get to breathe! Sounds much more exciting than "just being better", doesn't it? You will want to live each day with unlimited drive and passion to create, interact, explore and seek out any adventure your heart desires! From living these experiences you will feel ecstatic to be alive, grateful for every moment of blissful interaction. Your inspired emotions are compounded and built upon day after day, creating a cycle of more powerful thoughts that enhance your life. I am living proof of someone who has taken massive action on these beliefs and used them to literally change my brain and free myself from CFS.

Reframing the Stress Response

There is no doubt clinically that a maladaptive stress response is a major causative factor in developing CFS. The body and brain simply cannot continue to function in this state, and CFS in my case was the final wake up call to change my response to the stressors in my life.

The first step I took in doing so was to begin to think of my stress response as "helpful". It took some serious suspension of disbelief to view all of the awful symptoms as helping me in some way, but reframing stress in this way is a biological change that can improve everything. If you tell yourself "this is my body now helping me rise to meet this challenge", your body actually believes you. This cultivates trust and belief in yourself that you can face and overcome anything. After some time you will begin to realise there is no stress. There may always be stressful events, but you are separate from them and you get to choose how to respond. With this in mind, you can trust in your ability to handle anything.

I won't lie, it will take some brutal soul searching to look objectively at the fact that you are suffering from CFS and ask yourself the question, "how has it served me?" If you can begin to see it with a new perspective, you can begin to reframe the condition as something positive, as fuel to motivate you to find a way to improve all aspects of your health. Then you can take it a step further to become thankful for this impermanent affliction, as it has led to you taking positive actions to improve your life. This shift in your response will lead you to take even more positive actions and can have an amazing favourable effect on your biology.

Conversely, if you are constantly riddled with the belief, "I will never get over this", your body believes you and your disempowering choices follow—you don't maintain discipline in your diet, or you try something once or twice and give up because it "didn't do anything". These choices lead to emotions of despair and hopelessness, which then create a vicious self-fulfilling cycle as your thoughts continue to reflect your current physical and emotional state. This will perpetuate unless you choose an alternative. You don't have to be a Zen monk, but you are more powerful than you have ever thought possible, and you have all the resources within you need to heal. You just needed to be shown how everything links together so you can begin to apply your new knowledge.

To begin to condition a more positive stress response right now, you can practice how you will respond *before* the event. You do this by deciding on the type of person you want to be. It involves discarding the identity of the powerless sick person who will never be well again, and carving out a new identity for yourself, one filled with the conviction that healing and wellness are within your grasp. Ask yourself, "which thoughts do I want to have in my mind all the time?" and "which behaviours do I want to demonstrate every day?"

A person who deeply believes they are becoming well doesn't dwell on sick person thoughts. Your brain circuitry becomes wired to change by cultivating the emotional state before the actual experience. The physical and chemical processes involved in changing the brain through interaction with the external world

Reframing the Stress Response

are exactly the same as those involved when performing internal mental and emotional exercises. Your body doesn't know the difference between an emotional visualisation and an actual experience. This is why you have to emotionally feel wellness before your body actually does. You can literally change your brain and body just by thinking in a different way, leaving behind the cellular memories of the past and creating a new future. Changing how you relate to something changes everything in your world. Try and you will see.

Hold Nothing Back

Have you ever had an impulse to do or say something, but within a few seconds your mind got in the way, telling you it's not possible, or that you shouldn't? "If I walk outside to enjoy the sunshine I might crash from having to walk 20 metres and sit in a chair." This is an example of a situation I faced often, and many people with CFS also do, as even minor exertion can cause more lactic acid build up than a professional athlete experiences during a race. The problem with not following what your body wants is submitting to the fear of "what if?" The chemical reaction from having a consistently stressed emotional response means that minor activity *will* cause you pain. The not-so-funny thing is, because you're in this poor stressed state, the anticipation of, as well as the fear following any activity, will cause you pain. By practising self-regulation of your emotions, you get to control your bodily responses, and not the other way around. It's obvious to state that an increase in positive emotional experiences will decrease the negative emotions you may feel. But what if I told you the implementation of positive coping skills as well as following your body's subtle urges to seek pleasant experiences will train your brain to turn off your embattled nervous system's false alarm?

You can achieve this in a number of ways, but the key is consistency. The first place to start is to become mindful of your breath in all situations. Breathing techniques can be used to regulate and balance negative emotions, reduce pain and induce sleep. Stop right now and try this: Breathe in for 4, hold for 4 and breathe out for 8, keeping your attention focused on the breath entering and leaving your body. Remember diaphragmatic breathing. This simple exercise, performed regularly will over time, allow your mind and body to heal faster.

Other simple techniques to employ to enhance your coping mechanism is to simply say "Stop!" as soon as you become mindful of a negative thought. For example you may subconsciously think, "I'm never going to get better." Notice it, counter that with a "stop", and then replace with a positive, realistic alternative like, "Although I have this pain right now, I know it's temporary as I'm working every day on healing." Then follow immediately with a breathing exercise or something else that will give you a positive emotion.

Another key factor is getting all the crap out of your head that weighs you down and plagues an already challenging existence. You body is under so much physical stress living with CFS you cannot afford to zap your entire being of even more energy with unhelpful thinking, negative beliefs, resentment toward others or worries about the future. If it doesn't give life, don't give it life. So write it out, get it out of you; free yourself from mental and emotional debt. I have always been a people pleaser; in fact I have let people walk all over me, manipulate my time and force their opinions down my throat just because I was afraid to offend them if I spoke what was on my mind. A lifetime of living this way has meant I've never been able to feel like I could express how I feel. I supressed my own emotions at the expense of my health.

Some people are just impossible to communicate with. If someone has pissed you off and you're still holding onto a situation in the past you can't do anything to resolve, write an angry unsent letter. Even better, write the angry letter to this person then burn it. As you watch the paper disintegrate tell yourself repeatedly, "I am free now from the past." We can't go back and change the past, but we store emotional memories that affect how we respond today. For example, if we're suddenly faced with a situation where anger comes up, we draw up past hurts and respond with that energy. The best way to erase this burden from our body is to change our responses in situations now. As past emotions are stored until we create a new experience, it is best not to linger at all, but do something positive immediately. Repeatedly doing this will reinforce where you are now and will heal the energy from the past.

Another helpful method, if you can't resolve something, is to sit opposite an empty chair and envisage the person sitting there whom you hold ill feelings toward, and who has hurt you or made you feel unhappy. Yell at them in this empty chair. The brain doesn't distinguish whether someone is actually sitting in the chair or not. If you can resolve a situation with the person directly, do so, but being very mindful of your breath and your response. Your voice matters and you're entitled to any views you may have. Holding things in only poisons you and leaves you in a heightened stress response. You deserve better and by doing this you're showing compassion toward yourself. The body recognises this and will adjust accordingly.

It takes some effort to uncover what the body needs, as you are essentially trying to bridge the gap between the body and your emotions, and this takes practice. Something helpful to try and remember is asking yourself at the end of the day if you missed any emotions in any particular situations and failed to act on them. Persistently noting this and uncovering the truth of these emotions is part of the path to recovery.

With this concept in mind, a large part of CFS is not so much a lack of energy, but rather, it is too much energy that has become blocked. Specifically, it is emotional energy that has been blocked, which is then stored in the body. If this isn't cleared, messages are sent in the form of physical symptoms to alert you to primal emotions you have overlooked. You use a LOT of energy holding all of this inside! You have abundant energy – you're just blocking it.

Through a serendipitous series of events I was blessed to discover a method that enabled me to really put into practice concepts I was instinctively touching on to try and clear this blocked energy and strengthen my emotional response as a way of healing myself holistically.

Mickel Therapy

A lot of controversy surrounds Mickel Therapy in the CFS community, mainly criticism from those who dismiss its theories, haven't tried it and remain very ill. I think the main reason people are dismissive of Mickel Therapy is because the idea of healing something that is so devastating on a physical level by using emotional concepts seems incomprehensible. To suggest even the possibility of this succeeding almost trivialises the utter biological devastation occurring in our bodies on every level as CFS sufferers. There is chronic immune activation, neuroendocrine, metabolic and autonomic nervous system abnormalities, yet the interconnectedness of biology and emotional response is clinically undeniable.

I heard about Mickel Therapy early into my CFS journey. Like with everything, I tried to do as much research as I could, but as is the case with ground breaking treatments difficult to comprehend that you have to outlay money for, the details are often elusive. I read plenty of testimonials though – "I had CFS for 15 years and after two Mickel sessions, was cured"; and "I'm running marathons again now after 10 years in bed all thanks to Mickel Therapy." There was always a great big "BUT HOW?" missing for me, so I was quick to dismiss it as bullshit.

After another year of suffering yet very slowly improving thanks to disciplined diet, detox, supplement and activity protocols, I had progressed very gradually to the point where I could function at a minimal kind of level. I was able to be up and about hourly, could make dinner occasionally and could manage a 10 minute walk a couple of days a week. However, if I deviated from the plan slightly or encountered even the most minute level of emotional stress or upset, I was back to square one; in bed, in pain and with crushing brain fog. Around this time, Mickel Therapy appeared on my radar again in the form of the small CFS community I was in touch with through Instagram. An unfortunate fact is the chronic illness community on Instagram is in the hundreds of thousands, but I could only manage the energy to maintain communication with a handful. We were a small, suffering little bunch but were able to bounce nutritional, supplement and treatment ideas off one another and provide emotional support, as only we knew how other invisible illness sufferers truly felt. I am grateful for these people around the world and a few remain my friends.

One of these friends had fully recovered using Mickel Therapy after many years of severe CFS. She was able to succinctly explain to me how it all worked, and given that I'd spent a year digging within for answers, already changing and growing in every aspect of my physical, mental and emotional health, something about the practice resonated. After looking into the treatment yet again and discovering many thousands of CFS patients had experienced successful recovery, I removed it from my bullshit radar and decided I had nothing else to lose—apart from money, which I didn't have, as we'd exhausted all of our savings, tens of thousands of dollars spent on weekly supplements and tests. But if there was something else I could utilise to get me to another level again of self-healing, then I was determined to find a way. Well, the universe smiled upon me, because a week after I decided I was going to (somehow) start Mickel Therapy, we won just enough money on the lotto to pay for six sessions! I immediately emailed a therapist in the UK who came highly recommended and booked my first phone session.

Most Mickel Therapists I know about have been former CFS sufferers themselves, so they know what you're going through. It is also encouraging knowing they healed themselves from the "incurable" as well. That is the point most people overlook – *you heal yourself*. It's not like a talking therapy is a magical antidote where you have a chat and walk away better. That's where the bullshit radar kicks in and why most people don't bother exploring Mickel Therapy further. You are provided the tools, and then YOU must do the work. Within an hour of my first session I was filled with hope; not a false hope, though, like I'd been swindled by some kind of motivational pep-talk, but a hope through finally having clarity as to why my body was doing what it was doing and the actions I must begin to consistently undertake to reverse the process I was stuck in.

Throughout this book I have talked about CFS as being your body stuck in a state of overdrive. Referred to as the master gland, the hypothalamus is responsible for maintaining homeostasis in the body. This balance is critical for every system in your body, and when this balance is lost, symptoms manifest. When the hypothalamus becomes overworked it goes into overdrive and can stay in that stuck state. This theory is the basis of Mickel Therapy, which infers the hypothalamus remains stuck in this state. The hypothalamus is regulated by primitive emotion. The primitive brain is crying out to be fixed, having sensed vulnerability, pain, or limitations that have been running throughout your life or emotional traumas that have affected your coping mechanisms. The primitive brain will send messages repeatedly that something is wrong and needs to be repaired. It will remain focused on this until it is addressed and will raise everything to a stressful level to get your attention. As a result, chemicals flood your system even as you sleep and these actually work against your healing.

Lack of immediate response to symptoms can be taken by the hypothalamus as a signal you've done nothing and ignored the primary emotion. You do not need to live in fear of any symptoms – they are just the hypothalamus in overdrive completely messing up the homeostasis of the body! Responding to these symptoms positively will help eliminate them. Your body is not betraying you; it is getting your attention to change something. Through Mickel Therapy you learn how to interrupt the automatic patterns that are going on in the brain and how to replace them with positive actions that tell the brain you and it are not in any danger. By understanding and controlling the emotional stressors in your life and treating them positively, you will help your hypothalamus get rewired back to normal and begin to eliminate symptoms.

If you choose to try Mickel Therapy, I can only suggest you let go of all inhibitions and doubts and trust the process. It is brilliant in its simplicity, yet incredibly effective once you begin to consistently put it into practice.

The Initially Terrifying Act of Not Resting!

Living with CFS is painful and boring to say the least. Boredom and lack of fulfilment are often the underlying emotions behind brain fog symptoms, as we are repressing what our body really wants to be doing and not meeting our own needs. So how do we begin to listen to and act upon these emotional signals? Again, simply become aware and honest with how you're feeling and take a positive action, no matter how small, that leaves you fulfilled.

As an exercise to begin to remedy this, brainstorm all the things you really enjoy and are capable of doing and do them more. You will see improvement when you keep reinforcing these positive emotions in small steps. Something so prevalent with CFS, and I know it having lived it, is existing akin to a "Groundhog Day" mentality, where everything is the same – environment, foods, thoughts, emotions, limited activities if any – day in, day out. By noticing when brain fog is creeping in deeper and responding to that symptom by immediately immersing yourself in some small action that gives you joy, you are addressing this primary emotion of unfulfilment, and having done this, your symptoms will dissipate.

Another example of this is resisting resting when you have brain fog or pain, as these symptoms indicate an underlying primary emotion that needs to be addressed. This is the one thing that terrified me when I first started Mickel Therapy, and is a common fear for anyone with CFS. "I'm scared to overdo

Mickel Therapy

it" becomes your mantra, as the repercussions are often severe. However, have you ever noticed how strange it is that you are filled with anxiety and apprehension when you're about to go somewhere and do something, yet once *immersed* in the experience your symptoms abate, only to return and "pay you back" once the positive experience has finished? The fact is, the body is not paying you back at all, but rather, is craving more of those positive emotions and knows when you have slipped back into a suppressed state. This is not your natural state and your body knows that better than you do! So it's trying to jolt you out of this malfunctioning thinking-brain emotional state of overdrive to get you to listen and take action. You have to prove to yourself that the body never sends a fearful symptom to tell you to rest; it only ever sends healthy tiredness for that.

Something started to click when I first pushed the fear aside and tried this myself, and I can only say it was a miraculous result. Whenever I felt a symptom was causing that sinking fear that I immediately needed to rest, I did little things, like play guitar for five minutes, or walk for ten minutes, or go outside and throw a ball for the dog. I planned ahead for what to do next after these activities, rather than slip back into that habitual cellular memory of dreading the possible pain and symptoms that have resulted after exercise. Because, during activities, I was practically symptom-free! To me, this proved the theory that I wasn't "pushing through" or forcing anything, but dealing with the emotions of unfulfilment or frustration underlying the physical symptoms and taking an action to tell my thinking brain that I was listening to my body's needs and everything was ok. So chill out hypothalamus, you can begin to relax now! You must try to gain the trust within yourself that you won't crash and crush that fear. But if you do happen to have a "setback", you will be able to see why by linking it to your emotions rather than having "done too much."

Rewiring the Idiot Driver

Embrace the fact the body is not stopping you; it is helping you by sending symptoms as honest messages to protect you and get you to take action. Your thinking-brain emotions about symptoms will not help at all and will only exacerbate the flight or fright response, so it is essential you don't fear or dwell on symptoms. It is important to note here the contextual conditioning that may have taken place from previous negative experiences. To relay a personal example: I found myself driving to the shops on a day where I felt like I was ok. We CFS sufferers have these rare occasions where your head clears and your pain subsides and you think to yourself "Wow! Somehow I feel almost normal! I'm going to get out and do something." Well that was me, clear-headed and driving to the shops to get something to eat; a huge adventure for someone bed-ridden for a year! After ordering and sitting to wait, I experienced a sudden heaviness like I was instantly filling with concrete. I became dizzy and my flight or fright response sent me instantaneously into panic mode. "How would I drive home?" "I'm stuck here and no one can help me!" I got my food, made my way to my car and drove home like a drunk driver; foggy, dizzy and with little reaction time or concentration.

It was fortunate for all on the roads this idiot CFS sufferer didn't hit someone! Because of this occurrence, a conditioned response every time I tried to go somewhere alone after this meant I was anxious and worried my body would do that to me again.

Upon starting to recover, this feeling remained, and I was wondering why I was experiencing these symptoms whilst driving. Dr David Mickel states, "Symptoms are centred within the cells as state dependent chemical memories." I had created a negative neural pathway around driving. I knew I had to immerse myself in such situations where negative pathways had previously been created and create new positive ones. I had to constantly reinforce these so my body would trust me again and stop sending symptoms that something was wrong or that somehow I was in danger when I wasn't. By building new cellular memories with positive experiences, I've been able to increase how far I can drive and concentrate whilst feeling completely normal.

I would suggest also applying this technique to social situations or anything your CFS symptoms have caused you to become anxious and flee from, to forge stronger positive connections in your brain and calm your stress response. CFS is a lonely and isolating condition, and one where you really find out who your true friends are. Social situations can become non-existent, so it is essential you begin to recondition yourself to experiencing positive emotions again around like-minded helpful friends who understand. Do this regularly, but in short bursts, even if you can only handle 15 minutes chatting with a friend. You will be rewiring yourself to create new positive neural pathways that will become reinforced every time you make the effort to seek a positive experience. By taking action when a symptoms pops up, you are compelling the hypothalamus to start working normally again. All of these small actions are cumulative, and with attention, you will begin to see your symptoms are here to help you change your life for the better.

Listen to Your Symptoms

Listen to Your Symptoms

Symptoms are the solution to healing if we can uncover how. Traditionally they are viewed as pathology that needs to be immediately eliminated through medication, but this is a view that suppresses our true path to healing. Obviously if there is a growth that needs to be cut out, then you cut it out and move on with your life. When it comes to chronic illness, there is definitely more behind the scenes that require investigation. Symptoms in CFS are intelligent communication from the emotional brain centre to the thinking brain telling you what it needs to heal. You now need to train yourself to listen.

In its simplest form, many symptoms are the result of a primary emotion not being addressed. It can be as small as when you're watching a TV program and a symptom pops up, we often jump to secondary emotions, worrying and becoming frustrated about the symptoms. However if we simply tune in, address whether our body wants something different and take an action, the symptom will go. It's the same as when you're in a conversation with someone; they may say something you don't like, yet you suppress your emotion and let the person treat you unfairly by dominating the conversation. It may even be subtle, but you let it go and internalise it. This suppression is just one example of how allowing a behaviour pattern to proliferate throughout your life can lead to illness, and once at an acute stage, any similar situation leads to symptoms. However, by immediately noticing the emotion behind the symptom in this situation *now*, you can meet your own needs by immediately communicating, for example, "that may be your opinion but I feel this way…" disallowing that person to affect you and if need be, exiting the conversation. Your symptoms will go, as you have addressed your own needs first, and disallowed that dominant person to treat you unfairly for another second. You should never be afraid or ashamed to express how you truly feel. It seems so ridiculously simple yet over repeated actions, this has an aggregate effect in letting your body know you are listening to it rather than maintaining your old patterns of ignoring, suppressing and people pleasing to your detriment.

The body can be quite literal in the symptoms it sends to get you to address an emotion. I suffered a lot from tinnitus during the worst of my CFS. There were days the electrical storm in my brain and ears was so intense I literally wanted to knock myself unconscious. The relentlessness of it subsided over time, but tinnitus would always be the first symptom to reappear before an impending crash. After learning Mickel techniques and consistently applying them throughout my daily life, I began to investigate what the emotion might be behind this symptom.

A lot of my life I felt like my voice didn't matter, and because of that belief, I held a lot in, thinking people never really listen to me. So I started to reverse this belief when the tinnitus appeared, by always expressing what was on my mind, even if I had to literally say at the time I felt like no one really listens to me. To my astonishment, my tinnitus disappeared! So if you're experiencing the same, ask yourself "where am I not being heard?" Another literal example could be neck pain and the old saying that someone is "a pain in the neck." If you are experiencing this you may ask yourself, "*who* is affecting my emotions?" or "what

Listen to Your Symptoms

burden am I carrying?" Such concepts almost verge on the metaphysical. Author and all-round amazing human Louise Hay has established this path to healing before anyone. But I believe being open to and trying every possible avenue of healing increases your chances of doing so. In Mickel Therapy, symptoms have an *unconscious purpose* and it is your responsibility to interpret, identify and then take action to resolve the underlying cause.

The Switch Had Been "Flipped"

So what did I learn using Mickel Therapy on my journey to recovery that I can take with me throughout my life?

I learnt symptoms are produced by the body to get me to change something, to alert me to the fact I have disconnected and have become too caught up in my own head. Maybe I've been overdoing things or rushing or allowing myself to become stressed without realising. This is usually the case if I ever feel some niggling symptoms creeping in again like brain fog and lethargy. Symptoms are helpful and are a wake up call to take positive meaningful action. I have learnt my underlying lessons to change permanently, so as to avoid any kind of relapse.

I learnt to let go of all judgement from others about me, what I do, what I think, how I choose to live and at the core, who I am. I will never again waste time and energy trying to figure out other people's actions. I will never waste my precious energy with those who don't truly care about me or support me. Life is short so why bother? I will only ever surround myself with supportive and positive people.

I have learnt I must strive every day to bring new experiences into my life and to always embrace change. I have learnt to take action on my intuitive nudges, to listen to my gut and to feed my soul. I will always be on the lookout for opportunities for ways to respond differently, as this will lead to improvement with constant reinforcement of my strengths and abilities. Trying new things that make you feel joy creates more neural pathways in

The Switch Had Been "Flipped"

the brain. There is a snowballing cycle in effect here: the more you do what makes you happy, the happier you feel and the more motivation you then have to do more things that make you feel happy!

I have resolved to constantly strive for self-improvement, partake in activities I never would have considered before to build my self-confidence, and work each day to empower myself through positive actions. By varying my lifestyle and searching for new things that bring me joy, new places to see, sit and be and new emotions to consistently cultivate, I am constantly creating an improved self and breaking ingrained neural pathways. When you've been stuck in the routine of illness for so long, it is necessary to change all routines to create a lot of small positive emotional experiences. I feel amazing knowing I am breaking apart literally years of habits and stuck neural pathways. I know that slipping to old patterns of thinking and acting will create negative primary emotions like boredom, worthlessness and unfulfilment, which when left ignored, will cause symptoms to again shake me free from these automatic patterns of dis-ease.

I have learnt to trust that I will not "crash" again. Through my diligent application of this new way of thinking and behaving, I have crushed that fear. I know deep within that if I do the right things and live a healthy life on an emotional level it simply won't happen. If I do happen to have a slight setback, I am confident I will never go backward to where I was, as I now have the tools to address what is going on by linking the symptoms to emotions rather than having "done too much", and immediately move forward.

I will suppress nothing, challenge others and always stand up for myself. I will choose to walk away if need be and will always trust my gut instincts. I will remain true to myself and will always meet my needs because listening to myself empowers me with the tools I need to keep myself well. I have learnt to feel no guilt for meeting my own needs, because if I don't, I become unhealthy and if I'm unhealthy, then I can't be there for anyone else in my life I care about.

I have learnt to trust everything will be ok. I have survived and fought my way through a hell few would ever understand, except for those of you navigating your way through your own hell this moment. I will continue to work every single day in some way toward the bigger picture. I have goals and dreams to contribute to and change the world. To achieve this, I am constantly in the process of changing myself for the better. Beginning to trust in myself and the universe was a massive step.

I have been forced to examine every aspect of my life. I've learnt to ask myself and live by what I really value. I value my health, my self-worth and my mission to live a positive, inspiring and empowered life. I have learnt to never again allow toxic energy in my life and cultivate relationships with positive supportive people. I have learnt to let go of the past, worries, fears, hurtful people and focus only on what I want. I will never go into tomorrow with today's baggage, taking a momentary inventory at the close of each day to assess what I've given to others, where I've fucked up and what I can change about myself to make the next day better.

I have learnt to live in flow with the river of life, understanding and accepting that life is in constant flux and change. I learned to find happiness and joy on the journey to recovery, as life's challenges don't all end once you have recovered.

I learnt to have self-compassion and soften my attitude to

The Switch Had Been "Flipped"

the presence of negative or unhelpful thoughts. They are what they are and all things are impermanent, especially thoughts and emotions.

I have learnt to change *everything*. So must you. By breaking ingrained neural pathways, your stress response will begin to change to become more centered and relaxed in everyday situations. Simple ways to achieve this are by making small changes every opportunity you get. Try different healthy foods, sit in different places around the house or if you can get out, become a tourist in your own city, always looking for new experiences, sights and smells to take in. Begin to move your body differently, always being mindful of your breath and never rushing. You've been stuck in the routine of illness for so long, so now is your chance to change every routine you can possibly think of to create lots of positive experiences. Your brain and body will thank you for it in ways you cannot even begin to comprehend until you actually take action and do it. You will get better and better as this new way of living becomes a part of your life.

AWAKEN WELLNESS

Energy Vampires

We've all known an energy vampire. Become aware on an energetic level of how your body feels around others. Everyone has an electrical energy that can either empower and enliven you or drain and upset you. When you next spend time with someone, notice how you feel after they have left. Do you feel happy and relaxed, or stressed and depleted? Be honest with yourself. Of course you need to take responsibility for how you respond to situations, but anyone who leaves you consistently feeling drained needs to be let go of. You do not need people who stress, drain and upset you in your life, and you do not need to accept their unfair treatment or justify your decision in any way.

You matter, and your recovery (and life) is too important to waste your energy feeding narcissists and energy vampires. I've always been the type of person who feels everything on a very deep level. I'm intuitive and sensitive to the energy of others and have been labelled an empath, a trait not many understand and even I didn't comprehend myself until recent years. With this newfound acceptance of who I am and realisation of how I've allowed the actions and words of others to negatively affect me throughout my life, I will no longer tolerate or give energy to people who drain me. In this macho world, I'm finally embracing and understanding that, yeah, I am a sensitive guy, and that's ok! Life's too short, and I spent way too much time in bed to give my precious vitality to people whose negative energy I feel within seconds of encountering them.

Energy Vampires

Healing from CFS is about *you*. It is your struggle, your journey and your responsibility. It is your truth and you don't have to accept guilt, blame, inferiority or any other negativity imposed upon you by anyone. Your biology is counting on you to make positive choices. By truly beginning to mindfully tune into how your body feels and which emotions are brought forth from various experiences and interactions, you will find yourself beginning to own your energy and your power and heal your life. All of life is energy, and you get to choose how yours is directed, and what kinds you allow to impact you.

AWAKEN WELLNESS

Epigenetics

A core intelligence exists in every cell, and there is a part of you working on healing right now. There can be no scepticism about the power the mind is capable of wielding. In his book "The Biology of Belief" on the study of Epigenetics, revolutionary scientist Dr Bruce Lipton proposes that the environment of your perception can change your biology. It affirms you really are in control and have the power over everything in your life, even in this seemingly powerless state. To truly change who you are is to think greater than your body you are currently trapped in.

Along with your environment and what you feed it, beliefs determine your body chemistry. You get to choose how you live, how you create your surrounding environment and therefore, can alter the genetics of your malfunctioning body and mind. The consequence of a negative thought is equally as powerful as a positive thought, and you get to choose which. Why don't we all create a body chemistry we can flourish and thrive with?

In 2000, Nobel Laureate Candel found when a person learns a new piece of information, the synaptic connections in the brain immediately double from 1300 to 2600. However, if that information isn't repeated or if action isn't taken on it, those connections dissolved within days. If you can apply the information contained herein to your life today in some small way, you will create a new experience. Philosophy is reinforced and physically transformed into new networks in the brain. At this point, emotions are felt, and your mind and body begin to work in harmony. You are

Epigenetics

instructing your body on a chemical and physical level by acting on what your mind is intellectually absorbing. You are literally changing your biology.

Memories are stored on a cellular level. Part of life seems to be taking knocks and enduring trials and hardships as you grow up. For some, the trauma of past experiences may have led you to where you are now with your physical and emotional health. It was definitely true in my case. Sometimes we become trapped by memories of past experiences. We let these define us and live by the emotions these memories create. But this is not who we are. Those emotions are merely a record of the past and it is just that—the past. When we develop an awareness of the emotions we habitually experience based on what may have happened before, we can begin to let them go and retire the old self. In doing so we can begin to create an entire new self, neurologically and biologically.

How do we achieve these changes we want to make to heal and recover? The simple solution is to create empowering habits, such as those discussed throughout this book, until they become natural and habitual. You can change anything you want. You need to turn away from that "path" of illness. Imagine your future self well, on another path ahead of you, and head towards that. It's going to feel uncomfortable and unfamiliar at first, but all change is!

Practice, habituation and repetition will create a new you. Whilst I share my theories and experiences to inform and inspire, the real question is what are YOU going to do with them? Make your behaviours equal your intentions and your actions follow your thoughts. Train your body and your mind will follow. Train your mind and your body will adapt. It is only by *applying* information you experience positive change.

Meditation

"You don't sit to become a good meditator. You sit to become fully present for your human life and to develop equanimity, compassion and inner peace."
– Jack Kornfield

My mind is always racing. Constant light bulb moments and brilliant ideas to change the world and save humanity and what to cook for dinner for the next week and thoughts confused and confounded by the actions of others swirl around and around in an unrelenting chaos of light and sound! At least that's how I used to be. I'm still full of ideas and certain people's actions still perplex me, but now I'm aware it's all just what it is. Thoughts and emotions are like clouds that always pass. By allowing these clouds to pass, a sense of spaciousness is experienced. And it is in the spaciousness where answers lie.

I have gained a lot of insight into my busy mind and emotions through regular meditation practice and connecting with my breath. It's incredible what you can discover when all you're doing is sitting (or lying down) and breathing! I started to meditate regularly during my rest times, and times when I was just stuck in bed and unable to move. There are a lot of wonderful free meditation apps you can download as well as guided meditations on YouTube. You can also create your own mantras to mentally repeat whilst breathing in and out. A common example is to say

Meditation

(in your mind) "peace" on the in-breath and "love" on the out-breath. I spent some time practicing the following mantra:
(on the in-breath) – *with each breath my body and mind*
(on the out-breath) – *grow stronger and stronger.*

Whilst I now sit in silence for at least 30 minutes a day, these guided meditation apps and mantras I created became a lifeline I embraced every day. By strengthening your mind, you nurture equanimity, which, at its core, fortifies your ability to respond to stress. You then realise you are directly responsible for your thoughts and actions, and you are constantly renewing your resolve. That said, if you can begin to cultivate the feeling of certain emotions before you have actually experienced them, these envisaged emotions will be wiring new pathways in your brain. Practice feeling the empowering emotional states you need to heal, such as gratitude, inner strength, joy and resilience. If you do this every single day during meditation, chemical reactions and biological changes will occur that will allow you to bring forth those positive emotions more naturally in response to any future event, rather than your habitual automatic stress reaction.

All healing comes from within. During meditation, there may be things that come up that feel difficult and make you feel uneasy, but they are just thoughts and emotions. Emotions are only biochemical storms firing inside your brain. It's how you respond to them that determines where you go from there. Amongst the storms are the jewels that will reveal themselves to you if you listen. I always write any down as soon as I come out of meditation.

Here is one such jewel I found following a meditation in January 2014:

I felt like the condition affecting my mind and body is what is stopping me from living and feeling content. Then I realised I'm still learning new things. I work every day on improving my body and mind through nutrition, dharma and positive psychology, so in reality, I have great hope for my future. I must remember this when I feel all is lost. I will not be defeated. Though I accept what is now, I will work every day to live better and be better.

So sit, breathe and be. You may just find the answers you seek.

Emotional Freedom Technique

Emotional Freedom Technique (EFT) is a skill I learnt long before my journey through CFS. In 2002 I started to experience panic attacks. I was working full time as well as studying full time, and we'd just bought our first house and had a baby within a few weeks of one another! Stress overload! My first panic attack came from nowhere, and after a couple of months of repeated daily panic attacks I developed panic disorder and agoraphobia. Every time you allow something to negatively affect you, your body is instantly zapped with that energy and a stress response is created. If this isn't immediately dealt with, it accumulates, further adding to your dysfunctional stress response and hormone production overload.

I had been completely ignoring my body. I now couldn't work; I changed my study options to online so as not to give up everything and began trying to find a solution to the fear of leaving the house in case another panic attack hit me. The medical solution was to dope me with anti-depressants, but this achieved nothing. EFT was a relatively new concept then, and apart from learning how to breathe properly, apply cognitive behavioural therapy techniques and meditate, EFT was the main cure for my panic disorder.

Since this time, I have consistently applied EFT whenever I have been facing an obstacle, a new job interview or challenging emotional times to release the blocked emotional energy. I used it regularly during CFS when there were days I felt I was going to die and was terrified—such was the severity of my symptoms. It seems really weird and sometimes feels even weirder doing it, but is a proven technique and one that is now being used in schools to help children overcome emotional issues they are facing.

EFT works on the concept that emotions are stored as trapped energy in the body and that acknowledging and dealing with these emotions whilst stimulating (tapping) energy meridian pathways traditionally used in acupuncture can clear the emotions and the problem you are facing will be overcome. 'Tapping" gives you the power to own your emotions. Your flight or fright response was designed to enable you to run from a threat or climb a tree if there was a bear chasing you. The body flooded with chemicals in such an instance to give you extraordinary power to survive threats. This no longer applies, especially when you spend most of your days in bed as I was. The threats are now in your mind, worrying about what your body is "doing to you." You can no longer do the things you used to and want to do, so you are filled with despair, anger or frustration. Your primitive brain wants to fight. You also want to hide and find safety, and that is a natural reaction to the primitive brain telling you you're under threat. It wants to flee. Your body is trying to wake you up to something you need to uncover and address. It seems logical to want to escape the pain, but healing only happens when you tune in to your body. The cortisol chemical flood you are now experiencing must be re-channelled to healing energy. EFT can untangle that energy. EFT switches your primitive brain off and allows healing to take place.

You begin by acknowledging where you are right now in this moment, your present emotions and symptoms. When you tap on the end points of the meridians whilst focusing on your negative thought, situation or physical pain, you are sending calming signals to your hypothalamus to settle the flight or fight response. As you tap, the subconscious mind will open up further issues. Sometimes this may feel difficult, but trust any memories or thoughts triggered and go with them to explore further. You start tapping with verbalising the negative, and as you tune into the problem, you will notice a switch when it is time for you to begin reinforcing the positive with empowering and reassuring statements.

With CFS I delved into any unresolved negative situations I was holding onto in my mind, using EFT as a means to let them go. I asked myself, "when did these symptoms start and what was happening at the time?" I also tapped on limiting beliefs I had been given by doctors, parents and family, dissolving resentment and letting it all go. Through EFT I learned to forgive. The only reason hurtful people were still a part of my life is because I was thinking about them. I was creating it and poisoning my body. They were already long gone and cared not for my present situation. I knew it was within my heart to forgive and stop giving them power. Any situation where you feel you've been wronged or treated unfairly you can "tap" to clear the energy and let it go.

Consider the analogy of your child coming to you with a sore finger. You hold it, kiss it better; and it's better! The essence of EFT is acknowledging and accepting your pain or emotional distress and giving yourself love, comfort and compassion. Just doing this sends an immediate message to your primitive brain that things will be ok. As someone who verged on becoming stuck in the mindset of a life as a sick person, this tool became one of the most effective lifelines I was able to implement throughout my recovery. You can use EFT to dissolve guilt and blame, end self-sabotage and remove blocks to healing, deal with overwhelming emotions, overcome insomnia, heal relationships and so much more. Imagine what you could achieve in your life if you were able to apply an incredible technique that would interrupt the constant patterns of stress and limiting beliefs that come with living with CFS and thinking recovery is an impossibility! By lifting this veil, you walk even further down the self-healing path.

The Power of Expectation

I never once thought I wouldn't overcome this chronic illness. I had this belief challenged every minute of every single day throughout the years I spent in bed fighting to breathe, but I always believed that one day I would piece this puzzle together and recover. If your brain believes you *will* recover, it begins to settle from overdrive, allowing you to start the journey toward healing, as there is a reduced stress response. Optimism is crucial, no matter how overwhelmingly horrible you feel from day to day. The body has the ability to heal itself when there is a powerful expectation of recovery. If stress can gradually make you so ill, then why shouldn't an unwavering belief you are healing gradually make you well again? I have already delved into neuroplasticity of the brain, and from that logic, we can ascertain certain hormonal and immunological systems in our body, and therefore our recovery process can be controlled by thought and emotion alone. We get to choose our beliefs and choose our responses. Every response determines your body's nerve and hormone activity, as well as how your immune system reacts. Negative responses equal negative cellular activity. It is obvious then to conclude that choosing a positive response will initiate positive cellular activity. It is time to break free from automation and recondition new physiological responses to everything you encounter. By doing this you control your body and your health.

How do we create this expectation of recovery? There are many ways, as discussed throughout this book, to train yourself to respond more effectively in the immediate sense; mindfulness and breath control being just two examples. But for long-term altering of your ingrained conditioned responses and to reinforce the power that comes with believing you're healing, the secret is to repetitively trick the brain into thinking it is *already* happening. As I've mentioned before, the brain doesn't discern between whether a visualisation is a real memory or not. Any activity where repetition is involved, like present-tense affirmations and visualisations where health and vitality is your only expectation, create new connections in the brain that stay forever if maintained.

Repeating and conditioning new positive actions and responses will have an incredible healing effect on your immune cells and how they respond to stress. I found that once I began to consciously and repeatedly cultivate this form of imagined optimism, it became a belief, and I gradually felt less and less affected by everyday things. By "everyday things", I mean light, sound, talking and music; all ordinary happenings that would send a painful and immediate searing jolt through my system because I was so hypersensitive to all of them; they became things I could tolerate like a healthy functioning person again. My system was beginning to become more robust and my heightened stress response was diminishing. If you can begin to tap into the idea that emotional resilience and the power of expectation can block pain, rewire your brain and normalise your hormonal chemistry, you will find a power within that will make you feel unstoppable in your quest for healing.

Positive Psychology

Positive Psychology

Positive Psychology is an area I began studying once I had become functional again after wading through the pathology of CFS and felt encouraged and inspired by the progress I was making, delving into the emotional aspects of healing from chronic illness. It is a relatively new development in psychological sciences to actually change the emphasis from looking for pathology to looking for strengths and resources. CFS is obviously a pathological condition, as the cascade of malfunctioning bodily systems indicates, but there are inherent internal self-healing resources that everyone possesses and positive psychology can be used to unlock these resources to begin healing the pathology.

A tool used in Positive Psychology, as well as in Mickel Therapy, is that of creating a list at the start of your day. It's important to note, this is not a "to do" list primarily based on meeting obligations, but rather a list of enjoyable activities you'll look forward to doing throughout your day. Activity scheduling has a cumulative effect on well-being. Something worth noting as a CFS sufferer is the fact that some days you simply can't *do anything*; obviously, hiking to take in an amazing sunrise or going surfing won't be on your super-fun list. They certainly weren't on mine for a long time! However, there is always something you can schedule to give you a positive emotion, even if that seems minor or insignificant.

Feeling despondent because of your current ability isn't a personality trait you are destined to endure. It all adds up, and just by changing your "to-do" list, you will develop a new attitude, as you learn to practice prioritising positive emotions more. Some suggestions, which I did during the first stages of recovery, were small actions, like sitting on the grass outside, patting my dog, playing guitar for five minutes, listening to music I love, taking some photos on my iPhone, doing Qi Gong, hugging my girls and even dancing like a dickhead in the mirror to a favourite song for two minutes! By reading your list, your body and mind have something they look forward to. These are all seemingly trivial actions, but once scheduled, read first thing of a morning and then deliberately performed throughout the day, they are a deceptively simple method of, and one of the most effective techniques for, building positive emotions.

When you actively work on creating positive emotions in your daily life, you broaden your perspective, revealing more choices for yourself in mindset and responses. In Positive Psychology, this is called "broaden and build." The more you have the "broaden" mindset cultivating experiences, the more you "build" and change who you are. Ask yourself every chance you get, "what is an action I can take right now to show my body I matter?" You can literally help yourself become a better version of yourself! Increasing your positive emotions daily increases the key resources you need to live a happy and satisfied life. Your mental resources are improved as you learn to live mindfully, grateful for every moment. Your social resources also improve as you foster a greater connection with others. You will gain valuable psychological resources as you naturally increase your resilience and mastery of varied and difficult situations. Your immune system will also benefit from all of the above, resulting ultimately in improved physical health. This is what true healing from CFS

Positive Psychology

is about – acknowledging the connection between mind, body and spirit and using every possible resource to transform every aspect of you.

The Broken Spirit

The Broken Spirit

For every person who is living a life with CFS or has recently succumbed to its symptoms, the demoralising reality of loss gradually smacks you in the face with the cruel removal of every one of your basic functions and abilities. Initially you feel like you have the worst flu you've ever experienced in your life, combined with the world's worst hangover, and you begin to think "I hope this goes away soon so I can go back to work." Two weeks of this turn into four, then two months into four months, and you feel worse than you did initially, if that's even comprehensible. You can no longer work; that part of you is gone. The months turn into a year, and then one year turns into two. Your friends and family disappear, and those that remain offer hollow pleasantries. Blow after crushing blow rains upon your system and your being, as you decline further into the abyss that is living with CFS. You can no longer relax and watch TV, as a lot of people may assume we with "fatigue" must do all day! No, the type of pain where every nerve ending in your body is on fire and the malfunctioning cognitive storm makes this impossible, along with reading, writing, listening, talking on the phone, walking, sitting upright, turning over in bed, showering and for some, feeding ourselves. All dignity is lost. All facets of who we were have long gone, and mere shards of our former selves remain, evident only by the fact there is still a physical body of us in the bed.

For me initially, in this state, it was easy to succumb to despair. One objective look at all of this loss, and it was almost impossible not to feel as though my spirit was completely crushed. "What is the point of going on amid all of this scorching agony searing through my useless corpse?" The pain of limitation contracted my life to the point where I felt like it wasn't worth living. I tinkered with these thoughts several times, as I lay there alone most days, unable to move or escape this affliction. All I had been left with were my scattered thoughts.

It was with that realisation I set about turning my thoughts around. It was either that, or give up. I thought back to challenges I had overcome in recent years—I had coached my way free from debilitating panic disorder and agoraphobia that saw me confined to my house in 2002 for fear of stepping out the front door and facing the world. I then went on to move cities, play in bands and recording studios as a session musician and tour the country playing on stages in front of thousands of people. I then suffered a spinal injury and was told I'd never lift anything, run or play drums again, and to live on painkillers and anti-inflammatory drugs. I ignored that prognosis, did some research and practiced Pilates to regain my core. I also sought regular acupuncture; medically ridiculed but capable of permanently healing more afflictions holistically than any pharmaceutical ever could! I healed my back, went on to train in various martial arts, did regular sprint training and lifted heavy weights and bought myself a new drum kit which I now play every day! If I could overcome incapacitating physical injuries and terrifying mental illness, then surely I could overcome a chronic disorder with no apparent medical cure that had completely disrupted and annihilated my entire metabolic, endocrine, immunological, gastrointestinal, genitourinary, cardiovascular and neurological systems, taking away my ability to shower and feed myself?!

The Broken Spirit

Challenge accepted!

I knew I needed to keep my spirit strong, that my physical body would not heal in isolation and that I needed new thinking strategies that would awaken me beyond my physical and emotional limitations to heal myself from CFS and become the person I always knew I could be.

Healing the Broken Spirit

You always have your spirit. It may be crushed right now under the weight of what you face every day, but it is still present, keeping you here for a reason. It is what fills you with the courage to face another day of this, despite the pain and the fog. You may be feeling weak and lifeless as a CFS sufferer, but you are stronger than most people on this earth. You can become even stronger.

You always have your mind. You rule it, or it rules you. It is yours and you get to choose how it operates. Your thoughts determine your responses, which determine your actions, which determine your life. The strength of your spirit is determined by the quality of your thoughts. If you allow toxicity and resignation to flourish in your thinking, how do you think your inner self, and thus, your physical body will respond? The perpetuation of CFS symptoms is one answer. The continual weakening of your self and a latent inability to fight the battle you're in is another. You must choose.

I'm not special. I'm the same as you. I existed in a darkened room and needed help showering and dressing. Doctors told me I'd suffer from CFS forever and at times, I thought it might kill me. Had I not resolved to fill my existence with the combination of actions throughout this book, it may have. If I can implement all of these strategies to heal myself whilst barely being able to function, so can you. Great change never occurs from your comfort zone.

Healing the Broken Spirit

Everyone responds and heals at different rates and to different levels. Do not be discouraged by what feels like a lack of progress. CFS is a disease of three steps forward, two steps back. But as long as you keep taking those three steps forward, you will always be one step ahead. Be grateful for the small victories, for these will add up along the way. Write down in a journal every time you reach a new milestone in your health, and read over these on days where you may have slipped slightly. This will remind you of your progress and will remind you of your power to heal yourself. Remind yourself every day, several times a day, how strong your spirit is and how determined you are to heal yourself. You've got this.

The Art of Flourishing

We all have the potential to bring positivity into our lives, even though our circumstances may be an ongoing struggle. As I've mentioned, I was initially led to believe by my diagnosing doctor that I would have to live with CFS forever. For my entire life before CFS, I had thought a certain way, where my beliefs disempowered me. I had become accustomed to thinking of myself this way and being this person for so long, it seemed normal. It initially felt like my CFS diagnosis was just another nail in the coffin; just another thing that had gone wrong in my life. Something deep inside me knew this was my wake up call. I had thought, acted and lived in a way where I didn't value my self-worth for so long, and I knew from the day of my diagnosis that if I didn't change, I would indeed be in bed forever. So I dug deep within and accumulated the resources I needed to change, and began.

Every one of us has the same ability to find and uncover their resources and choose to take positive action. It takes courage to step back and evaluate your entire life and decide you want to change. It's definitely the scariest thing I've ever done! There is no one to blame for your situation, your difficulties or your unhappiness, least of all yourself. It is what it is. However, you are personally responsible for how you respond to it, and how you get yourself free from chronic illness. You must face the things you actually can change, and start work on those things immediately. This can seem overwhelming on the surface, causing you

The Art of Flourishing

to feel pessimistic, as it may have been a certain way for so long. So break it down into small steps and start step one.

Step one may be to give up sugar and gluten and change your eating habits. Or it may be to start your day with a guided meditation or thoughts of gratitude instead of dread. By taking the first step toward making positive changes in your behaviour, you will become better at coping with both emotional distress and physical pain. Your resources will grow, meaning you'll be more inclined to place your energy in what truly matters to you, exploring things the old you never would have thought to, and you will find yourself clarifying new values, beliefs and goals. You will begin to master the art of adapting, thriving and flourishing through life's transitions.

So how do we put into practice the art of flourishing? You should begin by listing all of your strengths you can think of. The old me struggled trying to think of any when I first attempted this exercise. If, like I was, you're riddled with self-doubt and feel you're devoid of any strengths, I suggest you kill that critic in your brain immediately. You are fighting a battle most people will never be able to begin to grasp. Just the fact you wake up to face another day of this hell makes you resilient, determined and filled with self-love. There are three strengths to start your list off with! If you have trouble identifying more, reach out to friends and family to help, as they will see things in you that you may not have acknowledged within yourself.

Take an inventory of your goals, dreams and aspirations, no matter how lofty they may seem, or how unreachable they may feel in your current state. Think of what you find fun and enjoyable and also the people you enjoy being around that make your heart sing. Imagine everything in your life is progressing exactly as you've envisaged, and begin to develop feelings of gratitude. When discussing the flight or fight response, I explained how our brain doesn't know the difference between a psychological threat and a physical threat. So when you give yourself unconstructive messages throughout the day, your primitive brain basically hears, "Am I going to live or am I going to die?" and responds accordingly, leaving you in a highly stressed state. The same theory applies when you're visualising joyful scenarios and feeling the positive emotions coming from those images. Whether you're capable of actually enacting the scenarios or not at present is irrelevant. The point is, your brain believes you, and begins to physically transform to manifest these changes in your life.

To reinforce the changes you wish to make it is important to write. In the worst of my CFS, I'd forgotten how to spell and was sometimes physically unable to sit upright and even construct a sentence. But when I could, I wrote, even if it was one barely legible empowering line that would get me through the day. If you can write, begin and end every day by writing three things you are grateful for in your life. It may seem difficult to find anything to be grateful for at first, but there is always something magical happening, whether that be the sun shining outside, or a simple loving glance or touch from someone you love. Hold onto these small moments, because they will get you through. You should also begin to journal any positive moments or events. Savour and acknowledge them, no matter how small or slight they may be. Any shift is worth noting, as you can return to these pages when you are having a bad day and remind yourself that the negative feelings can always be countered with positive moments.

It's imperative to begin to become mindful of your emotions and thoughts at times when you do have some clearing of the

The Art of Flourishing

brain fog, or are experiencing a joyful moment. What is your emotional state when you are feeling better? What kind of shift has happened in your thinking patterns? To what degree is your level of motivation changing toward applying the techniques discussed in this book and other self-care activities? Are you becoming more optimistic about your situation? Begin to investigate yourself and really immerse yourself in the moments when you do notice a positive shift. This will really help you to take on this new identity and enable your spirit to flourish.

Family

I cannot stress enough the importance of having only positive support around you, because you need help for every aspect of your daily life now: emotional, financial, physical and practical. The funny thing about succumbing to a chronic illness is, you get to find out who your true friends and family really are. All the well-wishing Facebook comments in the world are nice, but essentially meaningless when you can't even make yourself something to eat—as are the well-meaning family members who have no idea of the overwhelming dread you face every hour, filled with scrambled cognition and concrete muscles. They really have no concept of the gravity of the loss or the extreme nature of the symptoms, nor does anyone who has never faced this battle.

But there is no room for bitterness or resentment, as this robs you of energy you don't have to spare. It is essential you cultivate stronger ties with the people who really matter to you and care for you, and forget the rest. A huge part of this illness is learning acceptance, and in this regard, it is accepting that everyone has their own life and some don't want to be burdened with worrying about someone who can no longer do any of the things they used to be able to do with them. This reality might be a slap in the face, but it is true. What other people choose to think or do is irrelevant to you. Keep your spirit strong. People will try to make you feel guilty because you can't come to the family dinner or you can't speak on the phone for very long, but right now

Family

your job is surviving, managing your daily life and striving every minute to improve. Guilt, shame and people pleasing no longer apply so let these traits go.

I found I had to let go of my perfectionism, as my ability to do chores and function as a family member dwindled. I've always been the cook, school lunch maker, girls' taxi, ballet-Dad, karate-Dad, grocery shopper etc. With CFS, that me was gone, unable to even write a grocery list now or stand upright long enough in the kitchen while an egg boiled. That said, I was blessed beyond words to be cared for by my wife during my time with CFS. Although I spent my days in solitary while she was at work, I never had to worry about cooking dinner or taking my girls to school. I did lament the fact I didn't have the energy to do these things anymore, as I used to love cooking every night and being the school-run dad. Now my girls gave me a cuddle goodbye as I lay in bed of a morning and a cuddle in bed when they got home of an evening, as I was usually still there. I hated them seeing me like that, but I always managed to savour that brief moment of joy with my aching arms wrapped around them, and because of that, the fleeting minutes in which they saw me I was always smiling.

My wife drove me to appointments, was my voice when I literally couldn't communicate with anyone and washed my hair whilst I sat in the shower as I couldn't lift my arms. Having her and my girls in my life was my motivation for never giving up. There were times where I wanted to quit. I admit I did spend some days looking at my bedroom ceiling and verbally abusing the god who, if he wasn't going to help me, then at least could release me from this hell and stop my heart. I didn't want to leave, but there were times when the pain inside my brain and body was so indescribably overwhelming that I didn't believe I could cope with another hour of it. I always came back to my girls in my mind, staring at the framed picture on my bedside table and knowing I would get free from chronic illness and recover, because they were still here. Although I felt I was completely useless, I convinced myself they still deserved a father and husband.

So hold onto the ties with those you love most. Be open with everyone around you by communicating what your new normal is for now. They will either accept it and stay close or reject the temporarily broken you and abandon you. Either way, you can choose to resolve within yourself right this second that you will not be like this forever. And when you have recovered and are living an amazing life, you will not only have those that matter still by your side, but will be enjoying the company of new friends and acquaintances who better align and resonate with the new you. When you recover from CFS, you are never the same person. You become a warrior who has zero tolerance for pettiness and negative energy and will only ever surround yourself with those who respect you and lift you up. All else will fall by the wayside. Let that happen. Accept these losses as the collateral damage that comes with having fought the battle of your life by healing and creating a new you.

The Ocean

The Ocean

I am blessed to live 15 minutes from one of the world's most beautiful beaches. I used to drive there almost daily to swim, walk, climb the hill and train along the beachfront. Some days I would just sit on the sand and stare out, imagining all of the places I'd love to travel to. During the period from July to October it is not uncommon to see humpback whales breaching offshore in all their magnificence. It truly is a beautiful place and one I feel a great connection with.

It was heartbreaking to think such beauty was literally 15 minutes away and during CFS I couldn't get myself there. My wife would occasionally drive me to the beach to sit either in the car, if that's all I could manage, or on the hill, which I could usually survive for a maximum of about an hour. Some days the thought of even getting my body in a car was unfathomable. I felt every bump as a jolt to my nervous system and every flicker of light reflected from any object pierced by brain through my eyes. But I savoured those small windows of joy staring out at the ocean once more.

I don't know whether I heard or read it somewhere or whether it came from within, but during the worst of CFS I wrote in my journal "surrender your worries to the sea." There is spiritual, emotional and physical healing in nature and looking out to the vastness of the Pacific Ocean from Burleigh Heads on Australia's Gold Coast is my healing sanctuary.

You may live in the hills, the country, in a city or the middle of nowhere. Wherever you are there is ground and fresh air. Get out; literally force yourself to sit under a tree or put your feet on some grass or in some sand. Earth yourself. Earthing is now being proven to have enormous health benefits especially when it comes to reducing stress and inflammation. We are all part of this place and too often we forget our connection with the Earth as we're too consumed with our race to see who can amass and fill life with the most amount of shiny things. That's a race to the bottom and makes no difference in the end. The best things in life aren't things. The greatest difference you can make within yourself right now is to sit mindfully in nature, even for just a minute, and breathe and feel grateful, regardless of how you physically feel. Do this every day and I guarantee you will start to see an improvement in your outlook and your health.

Life in Increments

After about 6 months of sticking with my self-designed supplement and nutritional plan, I began to feel the fog lift and the pain sometimes subside. I had gradually progressed to a level where, on a good day, I could be up for two hours and down for one. If I skipped that hour's rest, my system would devastate me for days to follow. And if I experienced emotional stress or did anything more strenuous than sit upright in silence, watch some TV or do some research during that two hour window, again, I would crash for days with tinnitus and pain. For 6 more months this became my life; incremental periods of zero to light upright activity and communication, followed by a rest.

"Rest time" wasn't just a happy chilled out time in bed reading or something. It was a full blackout of all light and sound. This was necessary to survive the migraine onslaught and cognitive static. It was a time where I had to focus on my breathing counting backward from 100 to zero to drown out the anxiety that came with the mind-bending tinnitus and muscular pain caused by the emotional stress of being upright those two hours.

I used this time to visualise my recovery or better still, having already recovered. During rest times where I wasn't completely bombarded with pain and the light show behind my eyelids, I created vivid movies of myself running, mountain-biking, playing my drums again, swimming in the ocean and sharing laughs with friends. I felt these experiences as though I could go and do these things right now. I allowed myself to feel the joy one would feel if they were partaking in activities they love. I would then "awaken" to my entropy, still on my back in a darkened daytime room, the familiar ceiling weighing down on me. You might think this was torture. And in some ways, given my reality was far different from the fantasies I was creating in my mind, it could seem delusional. But I had hope. Hope is one of the most powerful things a human being can have.

My spirit rarely wavered. I knew from this slight recharge I could get up again and enjoy two more hours out of that bed. My progress was an indication I was doing things right, and I just had to keep going. I knew that eventually there would be no increments *unless I chose them*. Six months prior I was barely crawling to the toilet and wanting to die. "Where could I be in another 6 months?" is a thought I would keep at the forefront of my mind. This thought strengthened my spirit more and more every couple of hours.

Waiting to Live

What started as a never-ending death process had become a disciplined and repetitive regime of waiting to live. Any deviation from the routine with emotionally stressful energy caused a crash that could take me a month to build back up to where I was before. I was grateful to have progressed from the initial wasteland of acute CFS and the decade of decline before that, but I was frustrated, bored and stuck. I skipped most family outings unless my wife drove us to the beach for a picnic in my two hour window. Anything further required much planning, and at times I really felt like I was just too much hassle for everyone else to bother taking me anywhere.

One positive around this time was that I was getting my mind back. I was able to read and write again and was starting to have thoughts of what I may be able to do with my life when I recover fully. This felt like a long way off, so I decided I was tired of simply waiting to live again. I had to find something to do other than read about the CFS information, nutrition, biochemistry and research studies that had become the only knowledge I had been consuming in an effort to dig my way out of this hell.

Being a creative, I knew this suppression of my gifts in music, art and writing had kept me not only feeling trapped in my dysfunctional body, but also bored out of my mind! I was also broke, having not worked for a long time, and was starting to think of what kinds of things I could make with limited energy and funds to bring in some income. I screen printed my own t-shirt designs, and in my quest for home-business ideas almost started making organic soap to sell online! The possibilities really are unlimited now for people to create something and share it with the world, even with limited physical capabilities. All you need is an idea, an audience and a website hosting service like Bluehost.com that costs almost nothing and you're good to go! Now I had made a definitive decision I was capable and was going to DO something again, there was something greater I'd never considered waiting just around the corner for me.

Art as Therapy

I have always been a highly creative person. Growing up with a love of illustration, tattoo art and calligraphy, as well as having led a life as a musician since I was 13, were all characteristics of myself I'd since left behind. I had sold all of my remaining drums because I had no energy or muscular co-ordination to play them. I didn't have the strength to hold my Nikon dslr camera and sharing old photos with my Instagram followers had become my vain attempt at still feeling creatively relevant in the world! I was going insane and needed a creative outlet.

One day I had the (brilliant) idea of gluing my amateur photos to blocks of recycled timber and selling them. I'm aware a million other people have done it, but this was the limited extent of my original creative thinking abilities now! I was on YouTube looking for a way to coat the photo-blocks in resin and stumbled upon (as you do down the internet rabbit-hole!) a video demonstrating something called Pyrography. Somehow the interweb universe Gods had collided and interpreted me searching for 'timber, photography, art' and gave me an artform called pyrography. It's basically wood burning with special tools/ pens designed for the task. I became fascinated watching a Korean woman create the most stunning photo-realistic portraits essentially writing with fire. Something clicked in me and I knew I had to do this.

I did some research and within a couple of weeks had spent the last of my drum-sales money (which was literally the last of all of the money I had) on a professional pyrography set up. I bought some cut up pieces of timber to burn on from the hardware store. And there I sat, staring at a blank piece of timber (which is just as scary as a blank screen is to a writer!), not knowing what to do with this $400 pyro-machine on my desk. So I went and had a rest! After rest time, during which I spent a lot of time thinking about the Japanese art and tattoos which I have always loved and studied, I came back to my desk and sketched a geisha based on an 18th century Japanese woodblock print. I had expended all of the energy I was entitled to this day, but I knew something was kindling in me and that I would try again tomorrow.

And I did. The first lines I burnt with my pyro blade came effortlessly. I worked for 20 minutes! This was the longest I'd been able to sit and focus on something in a very long time. I had a rest and came back and did another 20 minutes. I was absolutely buzzing with excitement that I was able to create something again! Pyrography is a very slow process, much like tattooing. I had often dreamed of becoming a tattoo artist, but I felt my dodgy eyes, former back injury and a life of limiting beliefs made it just a fantasy for me. Needless to say, I loved every minute I spent recreating Japanese works of art on timber. The daily pain and cognitive dysfunction was so great, 20 minutes was the most time I could initially spend working. Consequently, this first piece of art became an intense self-imposed art therapy session over many weeks.

I gradually increased my art time almost to the extent that it became unconscious, as I was enjoying it so much—creating art and listening to music whilst doing so. Listening to music is another love I'd been forced to give up, as it felt like a drill in my brain. So I was happy and in the flow every day, listening to my favourite bands and feeling like I was doing something worthwhile that came naturally. My spirit was soaring from the cumulative positive emotions, knowing I could sit and create over increasingly longer periods of time. I remember thinking at the time, "if this is all I can do now forever, I'll be content with that." I had found some enjoyment again, and as a result, my symptoms began to dissipate.

Fast forward another six months later, I was recovering, driving my car limited distances, playing drums again, writing every day and feeling almost normal a lot of the time. Best of all, I could create a 10 hour pyro artwork in two or three days, and I loved every second immersed in the creative process. I was gaining recognition selling fine art Japanese pyrography pieces around the world, and had pieces hanging in the best tattoo studio in my city. Art, positivity and unwavering persistence had become my saviour and another piece in the puzzle to heal myself.

Gratitude

Developing a gratitude practice is one way to rewire the brain and enliven the spirit so we can relate to ourselves with more compassion. I say gratitude is a practice and not just an attitude, because it helps reinforce your conviction when you actually write it down and sit with the emotion. Start a gratitude journal and write three things you're grateful for every morning and evening. Advancing the practice another step, you will further cultivate an inner power by noticing how *you* made a situation happen that you're grateful for. For example, something I wrote in my gratitude journal is:

"I am grateful I created some art today. I made this happen as I pushed myself a little even though I felt spaced out. I ended up really enjoying it and felt better afterward."

Alternatively:

"I am grateful for the pain in my arms and legs I've been experiencing today. It reminds me to be mindful (as I haven't been) and to respond immediately with positivity to negative situations."

I read somewhere once that a good way to think in life is to remember that as soon as your head leaves the pillow every morning, be thankful you have everything you need. Well that's a challenging notion when you're unable to even lift your head from your pillow! I did try during my journey through CFS to become grateful for the smallest things, the tiniest improvements. I even got to a point, after regularly practicing living with a grateful attitude, to become

Gratitude

grateful for the pain, the restrictions and the daily cognitive challenges I faced as one by one, I saw them as being *on the way* to something brighter, rather than being in the way. It took a lot of reconditioning of my negativity bias to begin to feel this way, but as I did, I observed I began to spontaneously notice more things to become grateful for. And when I was faced with challenges, as we all will be, CFS or not, I was able to respond with a frame of mind that was more compassionate toward myself as I became thankful for all situations. Everything teaches you something.

Once you begin to truly feel grateful for the small things, it helps to savour that emotion in the moment. That means to literally just feel it and focus on it for about 10 seconds so you remember what it feels like to experience moments of joy again. Feel the pleasant sensations throughout your body. Even if something negative happened in your day, you can reflect on something you might need to work on within yourself or your response. Or perhaps you responded to such a situation remaining true to yourself, and therefore, you could feel grateful for the person you are. Remember, everything is exponential in every step toward recovery from CFS, so savouring these little 10-second moments of deliberate positivity really does go a long way.

Gratitude is the key to living an inspired and happy life. When you become grateful for the small things in your life, you begin to notice more things to be grateful for. Life with CFS can be horrible. But it is also an opportunity to be grateful for the transformation of every part of your life through self-inquiry and growth. Therein lies recovery. This is the hidden benefit of this devastating circumstance. Living gratefully encourages you to find meaning in everything. Once you begin to fulfil what's meaningful to you on a daily basis, you will gradually become filled with vitality.

Never Stop Learning

After some time I reached a point where I could listen to sound again. I had missed music as one would miss breathing and because all I'd read about for six months was CFS research, I was craving other kinds of information.

I constantly crave new knowledge and experiences. It's because of this I've never really had one "career", but many. Dozens in fact! I've played music, taught music, tinted windows, laid turf, delivered newspapers, manufactured tents, worked as a university librarian, designed t-shirts, worked in marketing, sold kitchenware, had a photography business, repaired school instruments, wrote and filmed a tv pilot, designed tattoos, did landscaping and wrote and staged plays.

I've also studied either at University, TAFE or online: theatre, English literature, education, herbal medicine, naturopathy, food coaching, life coaching, NLP, EFT, kinesiology, acupressure, mindfulness, reflexology, children's literature, photography, nutritional medicine, history, positive psychology, business marketing and music.

Now with my phone next to my bed and the ability to hear through the tinnitus and absorb some new information, I began subscribing to podcasts and iTunes university courses. I would lay there for hours learning about anthropology, history, exercise science, Spanish, classical mythology, justice studies, Buddhist philosophy among many other amazing things!

The point being, I was never going to submit. A huge part of

Never Stop Learning

who I am is this person who loves knowledge. When I couldn't read, I would ask my wife to read something from a website for me. When I couldn't see, I would listen to an audiobook. When I couldn't tolerate sound, I would write brief ideas, songs and poetry in my journal. I never once saw CFS as something that would steal every part of who I was or who I wanted to become. It tried to crush and destroy me! But I know how far I've come and will never allow myself to slip back, because I care for and listen to my body and nourish my spirit. Any little symptoms I experience now are just reminders to listen to my body, change something and take another positive action.

You may not be able to exercise your body, but you can exercise your mind, even if only for 10 minutes a day; fill it with something you love, something new, something old. Whatever you do, don't just lay there trapped in your self-defeating negative thoughts and staring at the ceiling. For the brief time in which I did that, it almost consumed me. There is always another way and that way may be something as simple as listening to an empowering podcast for 15 minutes a day.

It will lift your spirit immeasurably when you know that even a small part of your day is somehow fulfilling to you again. In the initial stages of CFS I felt essentially useless; I couldn't even feed myself properly or wash my own hair for almost nine months! But I managed to find new things from which I could gain some satisfaction. You too can discover new ways to enjoy life, develop new interests and find new meaning. When your gifts, abilities and loves are stripped away it is necessary to find even the tiniest fragments of joy again in your daily life. You must adjust, adapt and prevail, no matter what.

AWAKEN WELLNESS

Mindfulness

At its essence, mindfulness is being engaged and present in the moment from moment to moment, rather than stressing about the past or living in a state of reactivity. It involves focus, being present, listening more effectively and intentionally engaging with whatever we're doing in the moment, noticing when your mind wanders off, and then gently bringing it back to the present moment. It seems insane to suggest becoming more aware of everything when you're already well aware that you can feel the pain in every cell of your malfunctioning body! All of this pain and all of these mind-bending symptoms are real, though. Nothing goes away unless you face it head on, and symptoms usually persist until you figure out why they're here and what you need to change in order to clear them. Facing it; that's the only way to get through anything. With mindfulness practice, every time you bring your attention back to the present moment and out of your runaway thoughts is another moment of awareness. It is another small victory within yourself and another way you can heal your spirit, brain and body in progressive, manageable steps.

Mindfulness practise has been demonstrated to calm your nervous system and heart rate, improve cognitive function, maintain and balance cortisol levels, reduce worries and enhance gratitude for the small things in life. I have learnt a lot and healed a great deal within myself from my studies into mindfulness, mainly from the works of Thich Nhat Hanh, Jon Kabat-Zinn and practitioner diploma studies.

Engaging in a moment of mindfulness is simple, yet it requires effort to break free from living your life on auto-pilot and allowing everything around you to affect your emotions. You can practice literally anywhere (and you should), so here are three simple steps to take:

1. Focus on your breath. Diaphragmatic or belly breathing is your anchor. Focus on the sensation of air moving in and out of your lungs as the belly rises and falls.
2. Engage the senses. Shift your attention out of your head and focus on something around you. This could be a bird singing, a tree swaying, the aroma of coffee, the feeling of the sun on your skin.
3. Allow your thoughts to come. Acknowledge them and let them pass. Then return your focus to your breath and the environment.

I think the best thing about practising mindfulness as I was recovering from CFS is the fact it slows you down. I've always rushed at a million miles an hour with everything I've done, and mindfulness literally lets you go at a pace you enjoy and focuses you on being present. You're unaware of the impact your runaway subconscious thoughts have on your energy levels until you begin to live mindfully.

Here is a mindfulness insight I wrote following a massive crash:

I realise for the past week I have been pushing a little physically but moreso, allowing frustration and anger to sap me of vital energy. I must continue to strive for equanimity to face every situation with calm for abundant energy to remain intact. I must face my pain with mindfulness always to learn what it has to teach me. I feel like I'm back to square one physically, but I have gained this valuable insight from my current pain and fatigue, so all is not lost. My spirit grows with every wake up call.

Curiosity is the essential quality for deepening our engagement with our experience and bringing us completely into the present moment. We lose our childlike curiosity as we age, especially in this fast paced multitasking world, and the moments are lost. Our brain is on overdrive with CFS, yet ironically we're not taking as much in! So by bringing curiosity to the most ordinary every day experiences, we are returned to the moment. What can be more ordinary and something we take for granted as just "being there" as the breath? The simplest way to do develop this mindful curiosity is to focus on the breath for a few minutes; feeling it through your body, the rise and fall of your abdomen, the coolness as it enters your nose and noticing when you become bored and start having thoughts about what's for dinner or the pain in your legs, and gently return your attention to your breath. If you do this every day, morning and night for a few minutes, it will be a great start to applying mindfulness practice to more moments throughout your day.

Mindfulness meditations as a formal practice are just a starting point to learning to apply mindfulness in your day-to-day life through informal practices. It is pointless completing a 20-minute guided meditation if the rest of your hours in the day are filled with stress and worry from not remaining in the present moment. Informally applying mindfulness practice to your every day life means taking in the little things. You may like to have moments during your day where you set a reminder on your phone to encourage you to immediately focus your attention on your breath. With practice this becomes second nature.

Mindfulness

You should also begin to tune in to your environment and take in the sounds of birds, traffic or the wind, and with this heightened awareness you can begin to notice how your body feels. Is there tension? Is there something I can let go of? I found it incredibly difficult lying in bed with burning pain screaming through my arms and legs and trying to be mindful! In these situations one's mind darts around for distraction hoping for a moment of relief. I began to find with practice the pain would decrease because I wasn't adding to it with my thoughts. I was noticing it was there, accepting it wasn't going anywhere for now (or perhaps the next 10 hours!), then focusing on my breath and looking for areas in my body I could let go of tension. The pain was still there to an extent, but I could now relax into it by simply telling myself, "this is how it is right now." Becoming mindful in this sense affirmed within that I was no longer willing to waste precious energy fighting with myself. By generating self-compassion and acceptance that it is normal to sometimes have unpleasant thoughts and feelings, we jump less into reactivity and self-criticism and our alert system remains calmer. Stress is removed from the brain and new neural pathways can be generated in a positive way for long-term brain health.

I was able to take this awareness into many more aspects of my life. I notice how my breathing changes if someone says something I don't like – I can refocus and control my breathing patterns, returning them to a natural relaxed breath. I notice immediately if tension appears in my shoulders and let it go. I use the (formerly annoying) occurrence of just missing a green traffic light as an opportunity to just sit and breathe for three minutes. Stress dissolves and my spirit fortifies. I'm aware of my posture at all times and sensations like having grass or sand under my feet have never felt so amazing!

So by integrating mindfulness informally into as many moments as you can begin to become aware of, the practice will stop you wandering off into the default mode of worrying, dwelling, being caught up in judgements and self-criticism and not paying attention to your body. When "autopilot" or a dysfunctional stress response is constantly activated, your chances of recovery or relief from the symptoms of CFS are nullified. Because your entire system is already in overdrive as a CFS sufferer, the least helpful thing you could be doing is combining your emotional frustration from your symptoms as well as living in a state of distracted attention that today's modern world seems to command. Your flight or fight response in constantly activated and you lose energy and cognitive function just by not paying attention to the present moment. Conversely, when you learn and apply mindfulness techniques to your daily life, your flight or fight response returns to normal, your immunity increases, inflammation in your body goes away and your chronic pain levels will dramatically decrease.

Mindfulness will awaken you to what has been missing—an awareness and connection with yourself. It is yet another positive tool to integrate into your life to continue to heal all areas of your being. Looking back I can see I was meant to slow down, so that when life sped up again for me, I would have gratitude for every single moment of good health.

Wise Attention

Wise Attention

With CFS your energy becomes so limited your thoughts can be just as draining as a walk to the toilet and back. Thus, it becomes necessary to actively cultivate what is fit for your attention and what is unfit for your attention. Whatever you place your attention on is nurtured.

Happiness does not come from your circumstances, but your response and capacity to meet with balance and compassion for yourself, what is happening. It doesn't mean you submit and do nothing, but engage with this moment that right now is the life you're living. There is no other life in this moment so end the fantasy. This may contradict the notion of hopefulness and visualising healing, but you are freed from the immediate pain of wanting more and hating this moment. Let your loss bring ease in the mind. Freedom of mind comes from accepting what is for now. Although unacceptable, you're resolving to do everything you can to make right now better and happier.

From here, you begin to unify the scattered mind. The right kind of attention will bring you wisdom and answers. Through practicing wise attention, you begin to wake up from the trance of automatic thoughts and the emotions triggered by them.

Will we interpret this loss as so unjust, unfair and devastating that we feel punished, angry, forever and fatally wounded – or, as our heart, torn apart, bleeds its anguish of sheer wordless grief,

AWAKEN WELLNESS

will we somehow feel this loss as an opportunity to become more tender, more open, more passionately alive, more grateful for what remains?
—Wayne Muller

Qi Gong

Years before I became ill with CFS I was attending a free Sunday morning Tai Chi class at a local Buddhist centre. I was taught by a Buddhist monk and it was the wisdom imparted by him, as well as by the free Buddhist books the new local Chinese Restaurant used to give me with every take-away, that piqued my interest in Buddhism. I'm not Buddhist, but the philosophy and values have benefitted me in such a way that I now carry them with me from day to day. If only I'd practiced having more compassion for myself from around this time, I may have avoided all of the emotional stress I put myself through in reaction to others in the years to follow.

Qi Gong is similar to Tai Chi, but I have found it greater for cultivating energy. I have a good friend who is an acupuncturist and once he heard what I was going through, he contacted me and suggested I try a particular form of Qi Gong. He recommended Falun Gong and to download the exercises from their website. I looked into it and whilst some of the philosophies are a little out there for me and the video production resembled cheesy early 90s Photoshop techniques, the form is excellent for building qi/energy without much exertion. I practiced this form whenever I was able, and am pleased to say it did have a positive impact. Perhaps an energy pathway was unblocked and cleared in combination with the super clean diet I was enjoying. I eventually felt a lift in my energy levels, so much so that I returned to my regular Qi Gong practice for enjoyment and the ongoing health benefits of the form and its healing visualisations.

I highly recommend Qi Gong practice as a way to cultivate your energy and connect with your breath and body again, as this connection becomes severed in the daily stress of having to live with such a cavalcade of symptoms. Reconnecting with your breath and having compassion for yourself in all aspects of your life in all your actions and decisions will enliven your spirit immeasurably.

Visualisation

Elite athletes see themselves winning. Powerful speakers know that, once they walk on stage, they own it, as they've already seen it in their minds. Cancer patients who have visualised their tumour shrinking and healing with glowing white light have been reported to experience a greater chance of remission. The power of visualisation cannot be understated as a resource to help you heal your mind, body and spirit.

After a brief period of time hopelessly tormented by CFS and quietly swearing at my bedroom ceiling, I realised this was getting me nowhere! I recalled a children's book I used to go through with my girls that used visualisations as a means to overcome fears and worries. I picked up my notebook and wrote the heading "what will I be doing when I am completely healthy?" I decided there were no limits. I could do anything I wanted, and I wrote the list accordingly. Obviously, being bedridden for so long, a lot of my items involved ambitious escape activities, such as hiking, flying places, surfing etc. From where I lay, these things seemed unimaginable. But I had the freedom to choose to imagine and visualise whatever I wanted.

Go back to what you really love. What did you really want to do with your life? If you no longer have the job you had because of CFS, design your new ideal life. Even if you have no energy to do anything about it, you still have the energy to imagine, so when you do recover you can start putting those pieces of visions into place.

AWAKEN WELLNESS

I started to see myself in my mind as living the life I wanted to live right now. I felt everything as if I was in the ocean: the sun on my skin, the water splashing past me as a rode a wave. I felt the pounding of my feet on the ground as I ran along the sand up the beach. I heard the sounds the drums and cymbals made as I struck them. I felt the cool fresh air burst through my sinuses as I rode my mountain bike downhill through a forest. I could run. I could swim. I could play music. I could do anything. By feeling something as if I was already doing it or had done it, I was telling my mind, body and soul that these were possibilities and it was only a matter of time before I achieved them.

I began to notice changes as I sharpened my visualisations and honed my focus on healing my body by surrendering to a biological force that was greater than my thoughts alone. I knew deep within change was taking place on a cellular level from the conviction of my positive healing work. I certainly didn't start running, but I was able to walk for about 15 minutes without crashing the following day. I began to drive my car again, once a week to the library and back. I promised myself from that point on to delve further into the mind/body connection, knowing with certainty I would recover from CFS if I kept exploring this interconnectedness.

Visualisation can not only be used to create new neural pathways by imagined possibility, but also to manage and interrupt physical symptoms in the present. You can try this basic exercise that is based on Neuro-Linguistic Programming (NLP) techniques of visualisation to suspend and break pain cycles. It involves focusing on your pain and turning it into an object or a colour that you have complete control over in your mind with regard to its intensity. With practice you will begin to feel a sense

Visualisation

of power and control over not only your actual physical pain, but also your response to it. If you're anything like I was most of the time, you're possibly already in bed, in pain, so now is the perfect time to take action!

- Close your eyes and turn your focus to the area in your body where you want to change the level of pain.
- Feel into it, acknowledge its presence.
- Now visualise this pain has a colour, see it bright and prominent.
- Now turn this pain into a shape, you choose its size.
- See this object as being right in front of you.
- Now begin to drain the colour from this object.
- As you do so, shrink the object in front of you.
- While you watch the object shrink and diminish before you, picture your pain doing the same as you fill your field of vision with stunning white light.
- The pain is now shrinking to nothing, no colour or form, only brilliant white light exists.
- This light is where you can rest, knowing you have lessened your pain and its impact on your body.

This is an exercise you can do as often as you wish, and you should, to consistently reinforce that you do have control over your emotional response to what is affecting you physically. Changing this response will reduce the physical symptoms and remind you that you are not helpless and at the mercy of your body, but are still strong within and get to exert mastery over your perceived weakened self by consistently applying small manageable practices daily to improve.

Believe every day you are recovering from this temporary setback, even though it may feel like you will never be well again. Watch your thoughts, because what you think, you manifest. If you focus on this illness, you will feel this illness. If you visualise yourself in great health daily through meditations and have even a micro-improvement every day, your reality will change. You have so much power right now. Whatever you want, start seeing it all happening and it will.

Affirmations

When it came down to it, I knew I had two choices – I could be ill and extremely unhappy or I could be ill and happy. I had CFS either way and constantly causing myself mental anguish and emotional overload because of the severity of symptoms and the life I felt I had lost wasn't going to get me anywhere. I needed something that would change my emotional state in an instant. Still working with the theory that emotions have the power to either destroy or heal, I began starting my day with positive affirmations specifically written and memorised to change my state of mind regardless of how I really felt. It was a way to kick-start my day on a positive note from the minute my head left the pillow.

This is what I started every day saying:

I am so thankful that I feel so amazingly healthy, so full of life and joy and vitality. I have unlimited energy and my body feels awesome. My mind is clear and positive.

Yeah right! When you can barely speak or move, it's hard to convince yourself. But I said this anyway, and most importantly, I believed it was true, even if it wasn't. Your brain doesn't actually know the difference, remember?

By prioritising and ritualising affirmations daily to change your current state, you will gain more positive emotions, higher satisfaction with life, reduce depressive symptoms, have more resilience, become more in tune with appreciating the small things and will be in a better mind frame to plan for more positive experiences. Reciting affirmations every morning is about empowering yourself and prioritising happiness and well being as your natural state of mind.

I have included this list of affirmations so you can open to this section at anytime you feel you need a lift.

I empower myself to change things for the better.

If I don't like a feeling or situation I have the power to change it or how I feel about it.

I will use this temporary unhappy feeling I have to push me to take steps.

I always choose positive action.

It's an investment in happiness for all when I look after my own needs.

I will never be pulled down by negative energy. I am a role model for the positive path. I will lead the way and pull myself up.

I am strong and others are inspired by my example.

I will always keep charging ahead.

I will always choose to respond to stress positively.

I will follow my bliss and pour my heart into my passions.

I lovingly give and energy comes back to me.

I am so much stronger than I think I am.

I am emotionally balanced and strong.

I am filled with courage to express myself and be myself in my relationships.

Affirmations

I am experiencing a great transformation and positive changes which bring blessings.

I stay true to myself and trust in my own strength.

I always take time for myself and allow myself to receive all the good things that come to me.

I am always clear and honest with others about my expectations.

I focus on my power.

I have patience and trust all of the steps I'm taking are leading to the rewards.

I am guided and looked after.

I let go of conventional thinking and my divine life purpose comes.

I always follow my inner voice and make choices not out of fear, guilt or obligation but love and what pleases me.

I am always making steady progress.

I am always assertive and stand my ground.

I quiet my mind and receive the answers I seek.

I believe in myself.

I am brimming with energy and overflowing with joy.

I love and accept myself and believe I can do everything.

I am always protected through all changes and all things.

My body is healthy, my mind is brilliant and my soul is tranquil.

I can achieve greatness.

Everything is happening now for my ultimate good.

AWAKEN WELLNESS

I am the architect of my life; I build its foundations and I choose its contents.

I forgive those who have harmed me in my past and peacefully detach from them.

Today, I abandon old habits and take up new more positive ones.

I have confidence in myself and believe in myself.

I am clear and honest about expectations.

I allow my heart to be open to receiving love and healing.

I let go from a place of peace anything that doesn't serve my highest good.

I focus on my priorities and my purpose.

My ability to conquer my challenges is limitless.

My potential to succeed is infinite.

Everything I desire is within my reach.

I let myself go with the flow of change.

PMA

> *Don't care what they may do*
> *Don't care what they may say*
> *I got that attitude*
> *I got that PMA*
> —Bad Brains

When you're facing a crisis and it feels like there is no end in sight, you have two choices – give up or fight. In the case of a CFS sufferer, fighting is making your life manageable, learning all you can and putting that knowledge into action in small incremental steps every single day to improve the rest of your life! To do that takes the right attitude.

An impenetrable shield of light in the face of racial oppression, the acronym PMA in the Bad Brains song from 1982 stands for "Positive Mental Attitude." This is a mentality I've chosen to adopt at various times throughout my life, only to completely forget about it when the going gets tough (just when I needed it most!) It's easy to forget when facing negativity or hard times. So it takes discipline in not only thinking this way but also acting this way. In my case PMA now also stands for "Positive Meaningful Action." If something doesn't feel right, I can choose to do something positive that does. If someone is bombarding me with negativity in a conversation, I can choose to steer or exit the conversation taking a positive meaningful action step for my own peace of mind. If I'm unhappy in my work, I take a step to change something. I choose to create joy in my daily life and activities. Do something you enjoy each day and don't waste time with your precious energy on meaningless things. This includes negative thoughts.

One way to consistently implement this concept is to start realising immediately when you're feeling an emotion that doesn't resonate with your unlimited positive nature. Remember a time when you felt confident and assume that attitude in this instance. With diligent practice and repetition this new attitude will be your conditioned response in future circumstances.

Because I'm terrible at remembering things, I recently had "PMA" tattooed on my wrist as a permanent reminder to always strive for positive attitude and positive action. I can look at it right now and know I have the power to choose my state, my response or my action at any given moment. You personality creates your personal reality.

The Three Difficulties

"It won't work out." This is how I used to approach unknowns in every situation. I've always been a worrier. Now I'm a warrior! If worrying is something you're stuck with, there's a simple technique to break the unhelpful pattern that overwhelms your subconscious. It is training in something called "The Three Difficulties."

1. See and acknowledge your unhelpful patterns of thought and behaviour.
2. Do something different.
3. Continue doing that different thing.

It seems so simple it's almost insulting to your intelligence! But practice this habitually, and you will find the foreboding imaginary storm cloud lifts and you are no longer a worrier. As you practice, be grateful you're becoming aware of this worry-driven assumption and work to replace it with a more empowering optimism in your thoughts – "it will all work out."

Claiming Your Power

I spent a lot of my life not really liking myself or valuing who I am as a person. It seems perplexing, as I'm a nice person, I always help others and I've lived a life of variety and happiness. But for some reason I've always felt like I wasn't enough. So what do people who don't value themselves do? They sabotage their life, they remain in the shadows, they live in fear and they're paralysed to make choices. Recovering from CFS has taught me to value who I am, because I have endured, persevered and healed my entire life and therefore, have so much going for me. It is time to acknowledge that and live it.

So what do people who value their self worth do? How do they live? They make choices free from fear, they do things to benefit and grow themselves, they trust their instincts, they're not afraid to share an idea and put it into the world, they look after their mind, body and spirit and don't allow anyone who would seek to diminish them to do so. No one takes our power from us; we consciously or unconsciously decide to lose it or give it away. You have the power to choose your thoughts and actions and the power to direct your energy.

Where you invest your energy will give you a positive or negative return and every conscious thought and action is controllable and adjustable by you. The very nature of you being able to observe yourself thinking something unhelpful or doing something that hurts you is a leverage point for interruption and change. Recognise and avert this self-sabotage immediately by taking an action. Healing your life isn't something that happens; it is something you DO. It is an action; a skill set and gets better with practice. There will always be challenges, even after you recover from CFS. But how you perceive these challenges or how much power you give away during them is entirely controllable by you. There is always harmony or disorder. It is time to become mindful of always choosing harmony as if that's all there is.

Diary entry from 31 December 2013:

The last day of what has again been the most challenging year of my life. At times I've wished for death. I am physically disabled and endure the mental issues that come with CFS every day. It's horrible to contemplate but I've really struggled to cope with this at times. However, I've grown to appreciate what this has done for me. I eat cleaner than ever. I am letting go of past hurts and anxiety about things I cannot control. I am both going with the flow and cultivating a power I knew was always there but was afraid to fully embrace. I am trying to live each day with a positive mental attitude and allow equanimity and mindfulness to become a part of my being. I will grow more than ever in 2014. I will become the best version of myself I possibly can.

I may not be cured, but I will live.

Resilient Thinking

Resilience is a resource you can develop like a muscle you can build. It's not about sweeping away the negative, but *meeting* the negative with something positive. And it is a resource that develops and enhances every part of your being, as all systems work together for resiliency: your physical, emotional and cognitive well-being, your life purpose and meaning as well as healthy relationship development. The environment supplies all the stressors; you supply the coping method.

By training yourself to become resilient, you will find yourself better able to access your inner resources to buffer you from some of the pain and associated stressful responses that can be your daily life as a CFS sufferer. In Positive Psychology there is a way of managing negative emotions that help act as protective factors by increasing your stress hardiness.

When faced with daily stressful emotions, keeping in mind the "3 C's" will enable your brain to process stress in a different way.

Commitment: Make a commitment to reclaim your power. Remember, YOU get to choose how to respond to anything you're faced with. View your stressors as something that is part of a larger purpose and always ask what you can learn from them. When I was in the worst of my CFS symptoms every day, I always kept in mind the fact that this disease was changing the person I used to be from someone who reacted impulsively to everything,

Resilient Thinking

to a new, more relaxed and self-compassionate person. I took a devastating negative and chose to grow from it. You can too. Face this condition head-on with the mindset that it will empower you. After all, you are a warrior fighting to get through this day and tomorrow you'll do it all again.

Control: As much as you fight every single day, sometimes to just get up and have a shower, you have to recognise what is beyond your control and let go of the stress that fighting these unreachable goals or lifestyle conditions causes. That is the purpose of this book—to inspire you to take control of the elements in your life where you can actually have the most impact. These include diet, joyful activity, emotional responses, shifts in mindset and healing strategies. Everything else is irrelevant as right now, your full time role is transforming yourself to gradually heal and recover.

Challenge: Every difficulty should be perceived as a challenge and not an obstacle. Living with CFS is *instructive*, not obstructive. All of these things you face from day to day that you feel are stopping you from actually living are just on the way to you creating the most amazing version of yourself you possibly can.

The level to which you foster resilience within will equate to the level to which you will heal yourself. The sections in our brain that perceive pain and hardship actually assign and wire in emotional meaning to these experiences. Therefore, if you are in pain and constantly telling yourself "this is so horrible I can't cope", your brain immediately sends out stress hormones in response to what it perceives as a threat. If you begin to perceive the same circumstance with a different response, like that based on the "3 C's", your brain will not identify a threat and will emit an entirely different set of chemicals. Over time, and with consistency, this newly conditioned response will make it much easier for your body to heal.

You are resilient. After all you go through, you are still here reading this. Only those who are struck down by CFS know the true horror of what we sufferers go through. But there is a way out. The difficulties in life do not come to destroy you, but show you what you're made of and how strong you are. It will take every fibre of your being and the learning and putting into practice of things you may never have considered or even find a bit weird. But it is necessary. There is no single answer to recovering from CFS as everyone is affected differently. Do not succumb to despair. You must find an antidote to the emptiness of this existence. You cannot focus on outer strength, for outer strength is nothing without inner strength. Focus on inner strength and the natural flow-on effect will be an increase in outer strength.

So be honest with yourself. What kind of thoughts are you having that continue to create problems in your life? For me, it was the dread of having a body that "hated me", as my health problems in the years preceding CFS seemed to drift from one bad thing to another. The fact is, these events were only the outer result of an inner thought pattern and the subsequent actions I was taking because of that. I left it too late to realise I had the power within me to change these patterns in an instant. You have that power within you right now. You may be feeling weak and lifeless and filled with pain, but your mind can still think. And with your thoughts you can change your life.

If you want a joyful, prosperous life you must think joyful, prosperous thoughts! You are never stuck, as you can change your mind right now. Stay away from thoughts that create pain and focus only on what you want, regardless of how you physically feel.

Resilient Thinking

Tell yourself you are willing to release the pattern within that created this condition. Say it right now.

Release the past. If you're going to think about the past, only think of and remember the positive times. Sure, lots of bad things have happened in my life and possibly in yours too, but I'm sure you have good memories also as I do. So draw and focus on those. All of the negative things are events you have grown through and learned from. You are a better person from having endured and survived them, so remember *that*, not the constant replaying of the negative events themselves. Think only of what will make you feel happy in this moment. If your thoughts are anything but, change them in an instant and you will immediately change the way you feel. Practice this consistently until it becomes habit. Change your thought patterns now, permanently and with diligence. The thoughts you choose to think create your experiences. A negative mind will never give you a positive life.

You need to think about what you truly want. That's hard to do when it's clearer and easier to think about what you *don't* want! Most of my life I'd been an anxious and fearful person. As much as I've gone and done some amazing things, everything scared the shit out of me! So as I began to free myself from the CFS fog, I started to think "what if, instead of trying to give up negative, fearful, self-defeating thoughts and actions, I simply shifted or changed my identity and beliefs to those of an outgoing, resilient, confident person who embraces every aspect of life?" The result of making such an empowering decision would mean a person like this would never allow fear or procrastination into their life. I stepped into this new identity and do my best to live it every day.

Mastery

At some point, you have given up control of your life and your mind to others. You know your purpose, you know you have all the resources within you to recover and gradually heal. But it is your belief system that will stop you reaching and striving toward healing day to day. By feeding yourself processed foods, watching mindless TV, checking Facebook on auto-pilot and worrying about everyone else's perfect virtual life, you are allowing others to determine your emotions. You are giving away control of your life. Go within or go without, remember?

Start re-writing the script. NOW! Moment to painful moment. Eradicate "shoulda-woulda-coulda" from your life forever. Plan and apply. All second-guessing drains your energy in the present moment. None of it matters. Self-belief matters and doubt is eliminated through action. Unearth the beliefs that have held you back for decades and the patterns you unknowingly follow but don't even realise. Focus on your purpose and move forward. Right now your purpose is getting well and finding your joy along the way.

Start with how you breathe as soon as your eyes open of a morning. Then think of three things you are truly grateful for in your life right in this moment. Know your purpose as you get out of bed. Then make every tiny action that follows move you closer to your purpose. Don't react to stimulus and stress. You are separate from them and you get to choose how to respond. Plan for the future, have a careful look at the past and decide only the

Mastery

lessons and beneficial things to belong in your present. Cut and let go of everything else.

Have no regrets. This hell you are stuck in or making your way through serves a purpose and one day soon, maybe even in this instant, you will figure out what that purpose is. When you're in control of your mind, you're in the present. Your decisions have more clarity, as you're not reacting to external or internal stress and stimuli. You have a spaciousness between your stimulus and your response. You become the calm in complete control of your existence, methodically making good choices that serve you and your needs. You are on the road to self-mastery, self-healing and self-love.

Love is All

Life throws things at us to get us to learn what we need to learn and move on. Sometimes we don't listen, so the noise of life gets louder and louder until something breaks, forcing us to stop, reflect and take action to change, improve and grow. This is what chronic illness is for many of us. Why should we accept this? How do we deal with something that has taken away everything? When will we make it through this hell to the other side? I can only say you have to love yourself through your journey and trust in your potential and ability to overcome, for it is infinite.

I wrote at the start of this book that the only thing I was going to accept about CFS was that it was temporary and I would recover. What I didn't tell you was that I surrendered. For it was only when I surrendered that I began to view this illness as a blessing. Sure I was going to fight like crazy and learn all I could to be free from CFS, but I knew this journey would involve changing everything about my life, and part of me knew I had to just submit to that fact. I had no idea what I was in for—the pain, torment and loss—but I knew I had to trust this was all for a reason, and that I must embrace every step along the way as an opportunity to grow. I had to forgive myself and others to purge that negative energy. I had to begin to love and not hate the body I was trapped in and what it was doing to me. I had to embrace the fact that the love for my family and myself was all I had left in me. It was only then I began my transformation.

When you arise from the ashes of your former self, transformed by the weight of this journey, you will awaken wellness and know that CFS was a challenging gift.

>Through the Concrete Fog
>
>*I drift through the concrete fog*
>*Worlds away from where I once was*
>*But it doesn't matter anymore*
>*Nothing does.*
>
>*Stealing scraps of the sun*
>*I put them in my pocket*
>*For a rainy day.*
>
>*Capture a fleeting glimpse of*
>*Another day destroyed*
>*Wasting away.*
>
>*Sound awake*
>*Safe and aching*
>*Yearning for the light*
>*That'd better come*
>*So I can waste another day*
>*Stealing scraps of the sun.*
>
>*I drift through the concrete fog*
>*Worlds away from where I once was*
>*But it doesn't matter anymore*
>*Nothing does.*

AWAKEN WELLNESS

Nothing heals like love can do
Nothing does
I'll now forget where I once was
Because
Nothing heals like love can do
Nothing does.

Love is all.

—Dion Murtagh
July 2013.

Love is All

I Am Grateful for Chronic Fatigue Syndrome

I wrote this book to show people you *can* have a life after CFS. If only one person reads and applies the knowledge in this book, I will be both happy and confident they too will heal themselves from CFS. I do hope this book makes it into the hands of sufferers worldwide so they can become empowered with the knowledge and belief that their healing lies within.

I'm not 100% back to who I was, nor do I want to be. I'm a new me. I can no longer stay up all night and party or endure punishing weights workouts. I can't work 12 hours a day and I can't drive for 8 caffeine-fuelled hours straight as I would have in the past. But I don't want to. The old me who drank alcohol, lived on sugar and caffeine and never listened to his body is gone now. So is the former stressed out, reactive and anxious robot who functioned on autopilot worrying about the "what-ifs" of yesterday and tomorrow.

There is so much more I *can* do now. The new me, the wellness activist, lives on nutritious organic food, meditates daily, does yoga, Tai Chi and Qi Gong, is grateful for every moment (even the challenging ones), leads a happy and fulfilling life of writing, travel, playing music, study, creating art, hanging out with friends, creating content that helps and lifts others and exercises every day walking, swimming and bike riding. I still have days where the brain fog slightly creeps back, but it's usually only ever due to some kind of emotional stress I haven't dealt with effectively. I'm a work in progress and will continue to have that attitude forever.

When Aikido Master Ichiba was asked, "How are you always so centered?" he replied, "I'm almost never centered, but I know what being centered feels like so I'm always striving to bring myself back to the centre."

I live each day with the intention of improving myself or helping another in some way. I used to look through the slits in my timber blinds all day unable to move from my bed thinking about how great it will be when I'm "better." When you're committed to never-ending progress, *every day is lived getting better*. There was no single modality that was the magical cure for me and there won't be for anyone. Recovering from CFS requires an unwavering devotion to healing every part of your mind, body and spirit.

I am grateful for Chronic Fatigue Syndrome. I am grateful for every minute I spent alone and sobbing in the most unbearable pain you could imagine. I am grateful for being temporarily unable to read, write and communicate. I am grateful for the hours I suffered paralysed in darkness and silence, with only the drill ringing through my brain to keep me company. I am grateful my old life was stripped away from me. I am grateful for my journey through hell.

I am a warrior now. I have endured, learnt and grown so much nothing can negatively affect me again. I am creating a life I love.

You can too.

Thank you

My deepest gratitude goes to my caring chiropractors, my doctor, my Mickel therapist and the angels who appeared with just the right information and inspiration at just the right times. Thank you - Evan, Fleur, Gary, Mel, Saul, Rod, Bev, Sarah and Chelsea.

Printed in Great Britain
by Amazon